A WILD THYME IN THE CITY

A guide to **mothercrafting*** healing herbs
for cityfolk and herbal apprentices

MARGUERITE DUNNE,
Urban Herbalist

*Mothercraft: The buying, cooking, gathering, grinding, blending,
brewing, tincturing, infusing, decocting, baking, sautéing, encapsulating,
using, and mastering of medical vegetables, i.e., medicinal herbs.

A WILD THYME IN THE CITY

A guide to mothercrafting healing herbs for cityfolk and herbal apprentices

© 2024, Marguerite Dunne

ISBN: 979-8-35096-844-6 (soft cover)

Cover art by Kalena Schoen.

Dedication

Finding your own healing path is choosing a road not taken. Bushwhacking your healing path through the hardscrabble of a cityscape is a hero's journey. For people who've had to find their own healing path, this book can be a guide on your journey.

Many thanks to my students, clients, editors, fellow herbalists and writers, friends and family who have listened, counter parted, bedizened, and embellished my writing. There is no roadmap to writing a book, yet you have been my mileposts.

This book is dedicated to my father and his infinite quest for the truth.

And with a big bouquet of catnip for my angels Mitzi, Zolie, and Ra.

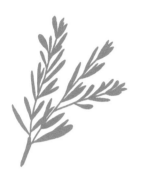
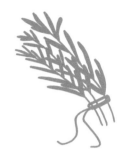

Contents

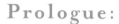

Prologue:

Portrait of an Urban Herbalist as a Young Girl

One of my favorite places to meander is the Dollar Store. For $1, my imagination is tickled into enriching my collection of kitchen gizmos, gaudily adorning a friend's present, or tripling my number of gardening gloves. This retail hodge-podge is fit for a Monday-morning writer's room on "Cavalcade of Stars."

One day, after stuffing my shopping cart with desk organizers, green and gold ribbons, and containers for on-the-road lunches, I happened to turn down the food aisle. A thirty-something, bedraggled mother, nearly a hundred pounds overweight, was towing three noisy, little children underfoot while carefully reading labels on soon-to-expire soup cans. She wiped the nose of the littlest one on his sleeve and scolded the hyper, eldest one, commanding, "Put those chips back."

She was just treading water there, a portrait in frustration. Not an American scene envisioned by Norman Rockwell, yet a true-to-life American scene in the cityscape today. Unsupported, overstressed, and undereducated about nutrition, this single mom was doing the best she knew how to do.

I remembered another thirty-something mother I'd met after doing an herbal lecture at a prominent health food store in an upscale Long Island community. That neighborhood had manicured lawns and children whose after-school schedules were more complicated than the flight patterns above LaGuardia Airport in New York City. This woman, who'd taken notes throughout my holistic healthcare lecture, came to me afterward and said, "You're living the life I want to live." She told me she still needed to get her family on the same page before trying anything new.

My college students often lament that their dorm rooms only allow them hot plates and microwave meals, so how can they eat healthy? Then I thought, *what if they were all taught about how to add good, powerful, medical vegetables—**herbs**—to what they were eating right now?*

Then I thought about the written questions I get at my herbal lectures:

- What's a good herb for energy?
- I'm on four medications for depression and still depressed.
- Recovery from a C-section.
- Chills and cramps, my period.
- Viagra's too expensive—some herb?
- Why do I sneeze every time I open The *Poughkeepsie Journal?*
- Waking up at 3:00 a.m.
- Herbs to focus—but my son's okay if he's building model airplanes.
- Why do they serve and promote milk in so many schools instead of juice?
- His tongue only swells a little when he eats peanuts. Is that bad?
- Keep memory.
- Back pain.
- Acid reflux.
- Allergies all year.
- My girlfriend lost 37 pounds on her diet, and I only lost 6.

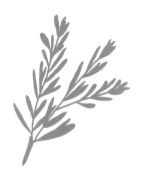
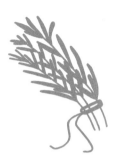

Introduction

A health issue becomes bothersome when it morphs into visiting doctors, a quarry-load of tests, and a shopping cart full of prescriptions. After leaving their doctor's office, newcomers to naturopathy venture into health food stores, look down long aisles of vitamins and health bars, and don't know where to begin. *All natural, GRAS, extracts, tinctures, vacuum-sealed capsules, powders with excipients, gummies.*

You come to a health food store to find answers about getting well. Those seemingly random symptoms in the body do tell a story. A small pain in one spot on the forearm, an ongoing sniffle, waking up in the middle of the night, and fidgeting are signs your body is speaking to you. These signs are telling you what is out of balance and needs healing.

Solving compounded, chronic health issues can involve false starts, dead ends, fabricated promises, and a stack of specialists, none of whom agree with each other. With holistic health, there is no one-herb-pill-fits-all because each person's story is different. Yet when the human body is understood, where to begin *is answerable.* It's beginning at the beginning and putting the pieces of your puzzle together. This puzzle is solvable.

Getting to the truth about my own body wrung a conflux of fortitude, second-guessing, research skills, grit, and trust out of me. I did discover answers, though, and some of them were thousands of years old; Mother Nature still prevails.

When my own healing journey began…

My dad was Puerto Rican, and my mother was Hungarian. I grew up in New York City, in the public housing projects with black neighbors relocated from the South, adjusting to city life, surrounded by neighborhoods of Italians off-the-boat, and Jewish people nursing wounds in the aftermath of World War II. The projects where I lived were on the East River, and every day, between garbage heaps and gang wars, I stared at the million-dollar skyline of Manhattan, which promised, and delivered, so many fortunes and adventures. I excelled at school, so was always placed in advanced classes which took me out of that neighborhood and brought me into contact with wealthier, more-worldly classmates. While I've invariably felt like my background had something for everybody, this multi-cultural, multi-class childhood did give me an odd kick to my gallop. It impelled me early on away from the idea of limitations, outmoded rules, and arcane, ingrained traditions that did not serve me. Even as a young child, I got to pick and choose from a potpourri of cultural values, guided by a heightened female intuition and honed through the crucible of the streets.

I first began using herbs in the 1970s, when, as a college freshman, the Margaret Sanger Birth Control Clinic put me on the birth control pill Norinyl, which led to painful leg cramps and a whacked-out endocrine system. After only seven months, I stopped taking them. When I stopped taking birth control pills, I lost my period, gained forty pounds, got a slew of allergies-including to penicillin, and began running 104-degree fevers. I saw nine different doctors: three medical doctors, three gynecologists, an internist, an endocrinologist, and a radiologist. Each doctor poked and measured me, siphoned my blood, surveyed my brain, took a stack of ex-rays, and prescribed shots and pills. At one point, they required I do a twenty-four-hour urine analysis, which meant I had to carry around a big glass jar in a plain brown paper bag to pee in all day. (Once, I forgot my bag in a college class and had to go back to retrieve it. Ugh.) There was no Internet with information-filled websites, medical libraries were only open to medical students, biology textbooks just described the names of bones and muscles, and the one PDR (*Physician's Desk Reference*) at my college was in the hands of a student council member who refused to let anyone look through it except himself.

All the doctors concluded for me, "There's nothing wrong with you."

I asked one doctor if, as a college student, I was going through menopause. Looking at the ceiling he responded, "That's a possibility."

I asked another doctor why I'd gained so much weight since I was down to eating one meal a day. He smiled and said, "Some people need very little food."

As a young girl, I didn't know how to respond to their stonewalling, non-diagnoses, nor probe for real, palliative answers.

Nobody would answer my questions.

Nobody would define for me what was wrong with my body.

Nobody would give me the steps to heal my body.

This medical limbo lasted more than three years.

Karmically, when I was home one night with my latest "there's-nothing-wrong-blood-work-report," my friend Richie telephoned. Through tears I described my latest, useless test and how I wanted to know what was going on with my body.

Richie simply said, "Let me take you to my chiropractor. He does herbs too." I stared at the pile of duplicated reports from those orthodox medicine men and remembered what C.S. Lewis said, "What saves a man is to take a step. *Then another step.*"

We went to see the chiropractor. He examined me, cracked my spine (which broke the 104-degree fever I was having), and told me which herbs to use. After just two weeks of herbal teas, I got my period for the first time in three years. Additionally, fifteen pounds fell off of me. That was it. I signed on the dotted line to become an herbalist and never looked back.

I got a few more gifts from that experience with birth control pills. There was an enormous sense of accomplishment, like an Olympic athlete setting a new world record, with paparazzi snapping away on the finish line. I hadn't given up. I had made it across that finish line when they told me that I could not, would not, should not try anything except orthodox, prescribed drugs.

(I would later learn that the birth control clinic had been acutely aware of its experimenting with my body. The closest I got to an acknowledgement of the damage done to me came in my late twenties. I'd moved to San Francisco and went for an examination by a new gynecologist. When asked about my medical history, I told him the tale of my missing menses. He replied, "Yes, we didn't know much about dysmenorrhea from birth control pills then.")

Growing up in a housing project, dodging bullets and gang wars, and fending for myself on a violent playground taught me not to accept any role society tried to assign me. After isolating myself from that torrid, outside world, I didn't have time to submerge myself in any tidal waves of grief nor retaliation. I already learned to set my own course and followed every new path out of that place. This birth control pill saga opened up a world of possibilities to me, and I was perfectly poised to discover what ancient herbology could do to restore my body to good health. No more letting health care facilities slice and dice me after another round of redundant tests.

At that time, there were still two, genuine herbal apothecaries in Greenwich Village, and I got to know each one very well. I began testing each herb one-at-a-time on my own body to figure out what worked for me and how it worked for me. There is so much to be said for that Yankee-know-how, rustic, pioneer spirit of carving out what is needed from the forest. And this was an old growth forest of knowledge, carefully passed down through generations of womenkind for nurturing and healing the family. There had

As Mahatma Gandhi said, "Even if you are a minority of one, the truth is the truth."

to be something both powerful and right in her-story to have lasted this long.

Herbalism is an oral tradition, handed down from grandparents to grandchildren, shaman to apprentice, curandera to novice, practitioner to pupil. When I began, in the halcyon days of innocence before corporations and backroom politics invaded the health food industry, I was lucky enough to be living in Greenwich Village, New York City, legendary home of bohemian artists, writers, musicians, and free thinkers. In walking distance from me was Kiehl's, a then 125-year-old apothecary, in the same building where it began in 1851. With my waist-length hair and hand-embroidered jeans, I easily strolled over between my college classes at Fordham. In those days, the Feds actually sent plainclothes agents to these bulk herb shops to ask questions like, "What's good for a cold?" If the person behind the counter said so much as, "echinacea," s/he could be arrested for practicing medicine without a license. So, while the people working at Kiehl's knew a lot about herbology, they would never disclose information about the virtues (virtues = what each herb can do). I found myself standing online at Kiehl's with people in their 70s, 80s, and 90s who'd all grown up with plant medicine. Resistant to the early 20th-century hoopla around the ballooning pharmaceutical industry, these elders had been raised on farms or in townhouses with home gardens; they'd always been treated with teas, poultices, and liniments. Their elders came of age in the 1800s, real farm-to-table kitchen-witching, growing up gathering, picking, pickling, drying, baking, sautéing, and nibbling on medical vegetables. They inherited the wisdom of ancestral herbology and, like their elders, were more than generous about passing this wisdom down. They told me which herbs to use when beginning a treatment and which herbs to use for concluding a treatment. When several herbs could be suggested for a health issue, they advised me to look for secondary plant virtues to mitigate accompanying problems. *The plants were giving me hope.* After my friend Ritchie noted my initial healing success, he bought me a copy of the original 1939 edition of *Back to Eden* by Jethro Kloss. It listed descriptions of over 150 herbs, all written with horse-sense, farmwife definitions. I began brewing each herb as a tea. I treasured this book for many reasons, including Jethro Kloss' description of his own journey from growing up healthy on his family's farm and then as a young man, moving to a city where he become ill. When Kloss returned to using his roots, seeds, bark, leaves, and flowers, the staples of his childhood, he healed. But even greater than this account of his journey is the 19th century sensibility he brought to each herb's description. That knowledge from the late 1800s, was passed down by his elders, and passed down from their elders, who were born in the 1700s. Over time, I've really appreciated this empirical Western herbal wisdom, honed and refined from about the 1770s to the 1850s. I believe this is when Western Herbalism reached its zenith. When reading the *materia medica* from this period, it is shockingly accurate for most of what is being written today, evidence backed by scientific tests, laboratory experiments, and chemical analysis. Crafted by nature, supported by science.

Blooming health is not a wild mystery to be solved. Ancestral voices, ancient gardens, gathered greens, and innate wisdom, were tools for avid apprentices and children assisting grandmothers and tribal shamen. Elders recognized the disruptions to the endocrine system without having cataloged a list of body organs nor even fathoming the components of a mineral. They understood plants. What had happened to me could be explained. There were solutions, albeit not written into the sanctioned manuals of licensed medical doctors, but passed down from one generation to the next, which included the deep, historic, intertwining of humans with nature. Humankind evolved having a symbiotic relationship with plants; they have always been our earthly allies.

An alterative and purgative, yellowdock sprouts up freely all over New York City. This plucky root has found its way to city lots and highway byways to imbue its spiritual gifts (releasing the old, decontaminating, and resetting the clock) to a population laden with disruptions and distortions.

Likewise, yerba bruja (herb witch), found in the coffee-growing regions of the New World encroached upon by civilization, defies efforts of eradication, by hand or herbicide, and strengthens the resolve of its mission, to alleviate hypertension. Mother Nature bestows these gifts on us when and where they will work for us. We need only to see and recognize them.

We keepers of the hearth, the nurturers, the healers of every family, the curanderas in every mountainous village and city neighborhood, we have stories. It is our narrative, the history of remedies and restoration, thousands upon thousands of years old. From sacred Eden to each urban metropolis, these are *our stories* to tell.

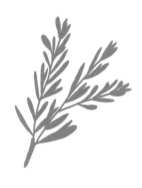

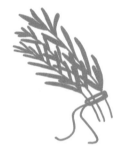

Chapter One:

Pulling Weeds

Herbalism, the Wise Woman Tradition, la curandera del pueblo

Ethnobotany began when all peoples were interconnected by tribal lore, had compassion for the heartaches of survival in an as-yet-undissected world, and with the ardent enthusiasm of children, carried their favorite leaves, roots, and seeds across the globe. History tells us that each marauding army appointed a physician-apothecary, attached to every fighting battalion. Trailing after the royal carnage, bandaging and repairing, administering potions and salves, he also collected species of plants from scared battlefields. Regimen doctors were taught about new plants from local wise women, who were still raising families and gathering from fields in between the bloodshed. These doctors made copious notes and conveyed precious samples back to the kings and parliamentarian rulers. In the West, some of our most cherished cooking staples were the serendipitous findings from the battlefield's edges: rosemary, basil, thyme, ginger, black pepper, cloves, cinnamon, and nutmeg, souvenirs of the Crusades. In later centuries, these herbs would deepen and strengthen the Eurasian trade routes.

The history of cooking with medicinal herbs is folksy, with happy stories, spiced with medical vegetables. Yet, the narrative of medicine has a coerced course correction, rewritten into the annals of physicians and 19th-century eclectics (the doctors who prescribed herbs, homeopathics, and newly emerging pharmaceuticals). Today, we are faced with a deluge of health issues, multiplied by Covid-19 co-morbidities, saddled with an allopathic Western medicine system directed by insurance companies who decide what will be paid for—i.e., treated.

In Renaissance times, the question for an herbal apprentice was, "In which meadow do I start to forage?" Today, the question for an herbal apprentice is, "Which book do I start to read?" bell hooks does a credible job of describing how *The Feminine Mystic*, Betty Freidan's ground-breaking treatise for changing a woman's role in America culture, was written about and for the well-fed middle-class-housewife who'd long been relegated to the diapers-kitchen-coffee-klatch-PTA world of the suburban mom. The turbulent 1960s found this housewife tossing away her knitting needles, eagerly competing with her commuter-three-piece-suit-asphalt-jungle husband. This was the newly-anointed women's liberation scenario; as the United Negro College Fund stated, "A mind is a terrible thing to waste." Yet, the ordeals of inner-city life, which have been endured by too many women of color, as well as the lower-income classes of European-American women, were hardly a footnote to Friedan's work. The upper economic class of women Freidan wrote for all found a way out or around any post-WW II limitations, and many went on to thrive when exiting housewifery to out-earn, out-curse, and out-sex their male counterparts. (Assertiveness training seminars were the rage in the 1970s.) I came from the neglected women's lot. Having grown up in the inner city, there was no time off for the luxury of ruminating on, "When I become a liberated woman, then _____ ." We were always working (as clerks, secretaries, maids, laundresses, baby sitters, companions, and several categories of sex-objects). It was not only bumping up against the low ceiling of expectations we faced, but there were also verbal patterns, holiday rituals, social norms, "niceties," and consociation assurances we needed translated for us, with no one available to do it. And after that leap of socializing, what about *our men* who were left behind? Was it a betrayal to leave them to the dead-end streets of dead-end jobs and crack dealers? Or was it every woman for herself? There was no ready escape hatch to be found, and the Friedan-inspired therapists marveled at the endurance records of inner-city women who managed to vacate that limiting life.

Because I was my own mixed-race, multicultural person and did not identify with a single group, I was entirely open to and ready for "What's next?" *Who can I learn from now? Which way is better?* It's been an advantage I've used all my life: not holding myself back because of others' limitations. So, when sipping herbal tea remedies was presented to me, I offered no explanations nor apologies. I followed my own yellow-brick road. In those early days, I became a lighthouse of information for those living the society high life of Manhattan, with aches, pains, and reactions pushed further down in the body by intense pharmaceuticals designed to suppress symptoms. When I started blending teas and making my own capsules on my kitchen table in Greenwich Village, friends asked questions, who referred their friends, and I began dispensing evidence-based information which had already activated so much restoration for millennia. Later on, I joined the larger, growing, health food industry and met other herbalists and alternative health practitioners who had faced their own traumatic health issues. It was through the ethnobotanical use of the simples (using one herb by itself), the medical vegetables, that our bodies healed, and our efforts equally validated our acquired knowledge.

Reading the Forested Cityscape

Beginning Today: The Toxic Overload

Concomitantly with jockeying up the corporate ladder, the women's movement grew in tandem with a back-to-the-land movement, which begat a reclamation of women's knowledge, in turn hastening the demand for organic foods, natural beauty products, and herbal remedies. Several generations ago, this would have been enough, but today we face a slaughterhouse of toxicants Mother Nature and our great-great-grandmothers never imagined:

More than 80,000 **chemicals** are used by **Americans in daily life**, and about 1,000 new **chemicals** are introduced each year. These **chemicals** are found in **everyday** items, such as foods, personal products, packaging, prescription drugs, and household and lawn care products. (May).

There are more than 7,000 chemicals in tobacco products, and there are more than 7,000 chemicals in cigarette smoke alone; more than 90 of them are linked to cancer (www.fda.gov).

- **Mercury:** Airborne particles, dental fillings, additives in vaccines. Health issues: learning disabilities, nervousness, personality/social changes, inflammation of mouth and gums, kidney damage, ungainly walk.

- **Lead**: Lining of the garden hose, lead-based paints, lead pipes, food contaminants, building materials, glass and ceramic glazes, used car batteries, leaded gases. Health issues: IQ loss, ADD/ADHD, cognitive issues in adults, nausea/vomiting, anemia, disruptive behavior, visual imparities.

- **Aluminum**: Airborne particles, aluminum cans and cookware, food additives, vaccine additives. Health issues: Alzheimer's disease, anemia, bone disorders, heart attacks, stroke, learning disabilities, inflammation.

- **Halogens:** Any of the elements of fluorine, chlorine, bromine, iodine, astatine, and synthetic amalgamates: Adhesives, carpets DDT, dry cleaning, herbicides, disinfectants, cleaning products, dyes, insecticides, toothpastes, swimming pool cleaners, table salt (chlorine), fungicides, prescription and OTC medicines (chlorine is used to manufacture 85% of pharmaceutical drugs;

Royal Society of Chemistry), paints, pesticides, water filtration plants, disinfectants, old photography development. Health issues: liver inefficiency, anemia, bone damage, brain damage, cognitive disorders, cancer, depression, diabetes, heart arrhythmias, high cholesterol, hormonal damage, reproductive issues, hyperactivity, immune system dysfunction, kidney damage, thyroid disease, breathing problems, congestion, tinnitus, inflammation.

- **Organophosphates:** Human-made chemicals to poison insects and mammals. These are the most widely used insecticides today. Used in agriculture, industrial farmworkers are at particular risk. Organophosphate pesticides are found in flea and tick collars, roach bombs, pest control sprays, shampoos, no-pest strips, insecticides, herbicide sprays, nerve agents, flame retardants (also added to plastics and textiles), powders for dogs and cats, and some fruits and vegetables. The symptoms of pesticide poisoning include headaches, over-salivation, nausea, vomiting, abdominal pain, diarrhea, rashes, miosis with blurred vision, incoordination, muscle twitching, slurred speech, cognitive impairment, and liver and kidney damage. In more severe cases, symptoms of poisoning include central nervous system depression (coma, seizures, and hypotonicity), hypertension, and cardiorespiratory depression.

Our modern homes also include dust mites, mold, mycotoxins, mildew, and bacteria. Artificial building materials, asbestos, latex paint, and lead pipes are still part of older dwellings and office buildings, garages, and public spaces, especially in older cities (May).

The Centers for Disease Control tells us six out of every ten known infectious diseases in people are spread by animals. (Witness the controversy over the origins of Covid-19.) Vectors are mosquitoes, ticks, and fleas. A person who gets bitten by a vector and gets sick has a vector-borne disease. Some vector-borne diseases, like the plague, have been around for thousands of years. In the United States, at least 2.8 million people every year get an antibiotic-resistant infection, and more than 35,000 people die.

The population of the earth is doubling at an unsustainable growth rate. The Earth reached its sustainable level around 1985. One billion people are now added every 12 years. One billion people who need food, shelter, clothing, jobs, and an active, interpersonal culture. There is no longer enough land for the Earth's population to live as hunters and gatherers. The resources to live today's "American" life, which the world's increasing population wants, are disappearing at an alarming rate. Organizations encouraging limiting population growth have not been able to get the word out, and politicians are kicking this can far, far down the road.

Taking prescription drugs has nearly become a roll of the dice…some 128,000 Americans each year die from *properly prescribed* medications. Prescription drugs have become the fourth leading cause of death in the United States. They kill more Americans than breast cancer, prostate cancer, homicide, and suicide combined. (www.nrdc.org)

The CDC reports that each day, 46 people die from an overdose of prescription painkillers in the United States (16,790 per year). Health care providers wrote 259 million prescriptions for painkillers in 2012, enough for every American adult to have a bottle of pills. (We now have 330 million people in American; these numbers have gone up.)

The National Center for Health Statistics (NCHS), at the Centers for Disease Control and Prevention, tells us that in the year 2020, there were nearly 92,000 overdose deaths involving illicit or prescription opioid drugs. Nearly half of the opioid deaths came from the notorious fentanyl, now being marketed in candy-colors of pink, yellow, and green to be pleasing to children. Fentanyl, a synthetic opioid, up to 50 times stronger than heroin and 100 times stronger than morphine, is often mixed with other street drugs. It is a major contributor to fatal and nonfatal overdoses in the United States.

The Centers for Disease Control also tells us that the highest week for people dying of Covid-19 in the United States was January ninth, 2021, with 25,815 deaths. The distinguished science writer Laurie Garrett, who wrote *The Coming Plague* in 1994, painstakingly details the origins of AIDS, the who/what/where/why/how it was transmitted around the world, the medical and political global response, and her final prediction that if humankind does not learn to live as an interrelated global village, we must brace for the coming plague. Covid-19 was not even on the map then, but time has proven her right. Nearly 30 years after her book was published, an identified illness "stopped" the world.

Political, orthodox medicine, which regularly makes hefty contributions to the Washington, DC politburo, doesn't always give us what's needed in preventative medicine. But a careful reading of women's gathering-and-ministering-history will. The ethnobotanical education that has been handed down (and validated by science) covers a core of knowledge about prevention and remediation for many illnesses and imbalances.

> People will pop pharmaceutical pills with all sorts of known side effects without a problem, but offer them something natural, and they become researchers.
>
> #bestfolkmedicine.

What/When/How Made Everything Change? The Flexner Report

The late 1800s saw the birth of the Men Who Built America (History Channel), and Gilded Age monopolists Rockefeller, Vanderbilt, Carnegie, and J.P. Morgan began directing more than railroads, oil wells, and steel mills.

By the turn of the 20th century, Rockefeller controlled 90% of all oil refineries, which had attracted experimentation and discoveries.

Not only was the world's first plastic created as an offshoot of the oil industry, but with an eye to the success of the newly discovered vitamins, Rockefeller recognized the opportunity to produce chemicals and medicines from his monopoly. Yet Rockefeller knew he was facing a hard sell, since herbal remedies were still widely used and accepted in America. "Almost half the doctors and medical colleges in the U.S. were practicing holistic medicine, using knowledge from Europe and Native Americans." (Rockefeller-Founded-Big-Pharma) Faced with the classic business dilemma of "problem–reaction–solution," Rockefeller went to Carnegie to create a problem with a pre-planned solution to follow not far behind. The Carnegie Foundation sent out Abraham Flexner to travel around the States visiting medical colleges and hospitals "to ascertain" the state of the art of medicine. (Rockefeller-Founded-Big-Pharma)

"In the early 1900s, the Carnegie Foundation and the American Medical Association tasked Abraham Flexner, an education specialist, with traveling to all 155 medical schools in the U.S. and Canada to assess the state of medical education." (Medpage Today)

"The Flexner Report" is a book-length landmark report of medical education in the United States and Canada, published in 1910 under the aegis of the Carnegie Foundation.

"The Flexner Report of 1910 transformed the nature and process of medical education in America, with a resulting elimination of proprietary schools and the establishment of the biomedical model as the good standard of medical training. This transformation occurred in the aftermath of the report, which embraced scientific knowledge and its advancement as the defining ethos of a modern physician. Such an orientation had its origins in the enchantment with German medical education that was spurred at the turn of the century by the exposure of American educators and physicians to the university medical schools of Europe. American medicine profited immeasurably from the scientific advances that this system allowed, but the hyper-rational system of German science created an imbalance in the art and science of medicine." (The National Library of Medicine)

"The Flexner Report (also called Carnegie Foundation Bulletin Number Four) called on American medical schools to enact exacting academic admission and graduation standards, and to adhere strictly to the protocols of mainstream, institutionalized science in teaching and research. Many American medical schools fell short of the standards advocated in the Flexner Report, and subsequent to its publication, nearly half of such schools merged or were closed outright." (Wikipedia)

Homeopathy, osteopathy, eclectic medicine, and physiomedicalism (botanical therapies that had not been tested according to the orthodox standards used for drugs) were derided. Some doctors were jailed.

The Report also concluded that there were too many medical school in the United States, training too many doctors. A sad repercussion of the Report was the reversion back to male-only admittance programs, effectively creating a smaller admission pool. (Universities had really begun expanding female admissions for women's and co-educational facilities in the mid-to-latter part of the 19th century with co-educational Oberlin College and private women's colleges such as Vassar and Pembroke.) (Wikipedia)

"To help with the transition and change the minds of other doctors and scientists, Rockefeller gave more than $100 million to colleges [and] hospitals, and founded a philanthropic front group called 'General Education Board' (GEB). This is the classic carrot and stick approach. In a very short time, medical colleges were all streamlined and homogenized. All the students were learning the same thing, and medicine was all about using patented drugs." (Rockefeller-Founded-Big-Pharma)

Black Medical Schools

"No single document on medical education had more impact on the training of physicians that the Flexner Report on Medical education in the United States and Canada...Close scrutiny of Flexner's two-page chapter on black medical education in this unique report provokes thought about the long-term effect on medical education for blacks...In 1901, the AMA voiced objections to the quality of care provided to Americans and began to criticize medical education. Because of a surplus of ineffective practitioners, the AMA formed the Council on Medical Education (CME) to determine the future of medical education...The Carnegie Foundation for the Advancement of Teaching agreed to undertake the task and selected an educator, Abraham Flexner, to conduct the separate inquiry. Flexner began his study with the medical school at Johns Hopkins because the institution was considered to be the pinnacle of U.S. medical education. Using Johns Hopkins as the standard, Flexner visited 155 medical schools and made observations on admissions requirements, size and credentials of faculty, endowment funds, student fees, quality of instruction in the classroom, laboratories, and clinics, and the relationship between the medical schools and their hospital affiliates... 'The medical care of the negro race will never be wholly left to negro physicians. Nevertheless, if the negro can be brought to feel a sharp responsibility for the physical integrity of his people, the outlook for their mental and moral improvement will be distinctly brightened. But the physical well-being of the negro is not only of the moment to the negro himself. Ten million of them live in close contact with 60 million whites. Not only does the negro himself suffer from hookworm and tuberculosis, he communicates them to his white neighbors, precisely as the ignorant and unfortunate white which contaminates him... The pioneer work in educating the race to know and to practice fundamental hygienic principles must be done largely by the negro physician and the negro nurse. It is important that they both be sensibly and effectively trained at the level at which their services are now important...The negro needs good schools rather than many schools-schools to which the more promising of the race can be sent to receive a substantial education in which hygiene rather that surgery, for example, is strongly accentuated. If at the same time these men can be imbued with the missionary spirit so that they will look upon the diploma as a commission to service their people humbly and devotedly, they may play an important part in the sanitation and civilization of the whole nation. Their duty calls them away from large cities to the village and the plantation, upon which light has hardly as yet begun to break...Meharry at Nashville and Howard at Washington [medical schools] are worth developing, and until considerably increased benefactions are available, effort will wisely concentrate upon them. [Note: Five other black medical colleges were closed because of Flexner's findings.]. The future of Howard is assured; indeed, the new Freedman's Hospital is an asset the like of which is in this country extremely rare. It is greatly to be hoped that the government may display a liberal and progressive spirit in adapting the administration of this institution to the requirement of medical education...'

Flexner's recommendation was for black medical students to focus on basic principles of health and hygiene. The implication was to restrict blacks to an elementary form of practice. Without access to surgery and research, black medical practice would be confined to rudimentary tasks. Consequently, Flexner's statement served to hinder black physicians in the pursuit of more sophisticated endeavors..." (The Flexner Report and Black Academic Medicine: An Assignment of Place Https://www.ncbi.nlm.nih.gov/pmc/articles/PMC2571842/pdf/jnma00292-0091.pdf)

Allegedly looking "to focus" the efforts of African-American medical professionals, black medical schools were less about advanced studies and more about hygiene. Again, the weight of this report was limiting whatever empirical, ethnobotanical, and scientific knowledge may have developed or which was already in use by active practitioners.

It is known that when Africans were enslaved and brought to the New World, they often spent their evenings hunting and gathering in the forests for their own food and medicines. Accustomed to the ethnobotany of Africa, they did develop their own vibrant, nursing systems and healing remedies. They had to survive. With the advent of the Flexner report's influence, this additional information was largely left by the wayside along with many promising eager, bright African-American students who were ready to be fully trained as educated doctors.

The National Library of Medicine, under the National Institutes of Health and the Carnegie Institute, detailed the training, steps, and European collegiate educational standards, which influenced the seismic shift in the American medical model at that time. Additionally, the advents of telephones, the transatlantic cable, the expansion of skyscrapers, the spreading of industrial parks thanks to pedestrian and automobile traffic, and the greater cultural influence of moving pictures all conspired to alter the consciousness from farmstead life to decided cosmopolitan choices. "Homemade" remedies and salves were seen as "hickish," and the Jazz Age became the talk of the town. "[Botanicals and their products which were already] in the USP (United States Pharmacopeia) became a wedge issue used by the AMA (American Medical Association) to express disdain with the USP revision process, which the AMA believed should be in the control of physicians rather than pharmacists. From 1900 to 1910, all USP revision committee members were pharmacists. By 1909, a report issued by an ad hoc Committee on the Revision of the Pharmacopeia of the American Medical Association (not to be confused with USP's official revision convention) lobbied to have (more than 40 additional botanicals) removed from the USP." (Herbalgram) The award-winning author, investigative journalist, and filmmaker Kenny Ausubel won the prestigious "Best Censored Stories" journalism award for his acclaimed documentary on the Harry Hoxsey case. In his brilliant book, *When Healing Becomes a Crime,* Ausubel details the story of fourth-generation herbalist Harry Hoxsey whose herbal formula successfully treated thousands for cancer in the early 1900s. (It had been passed down in his family since the mid-1800s.) At one point, Hoxsey had clinics in 17 states and his own radio show. The AMA's Morris Fishbein (who never practiced medicine a day in his life) wanted to buy the formula to be marketed under the aegis of the AMA. However, negotiations with Hoxsey broke down over the Quaker Hoxsey family tradition of giving away the formula for free if someone could not afford to pay for it. Hoxsey pulled out of the deal and the AMA went on the warpath. Hoxsey was arrested more than 50 times and sued dozens of times (he always won because so many positive witnesses testified for him). Eventually, Hoxsey was personally bankrupt and worn out. He closed his American clinics. (The elaborate particulars of this intriguing saga are itemized in Ausubel's book.)

After the Flexner Report, as Carnegie and Rockefeller invested in Big Pharma, and distribution of information about the efficacy of herbs slowed down. The oral-herbal tradition, invalidated and much pooh-poohed, went underground.

Herbalism had been passed down from grandmother to grand-daughter. Women went to the creek and washed their family's clothes, traded botanical recipes, and talked about birthing, babies, swaddling, sniffles, mending broken bones, the deep scars of chicken pox, sewing a hunter's flesh wounds after bear attacks, recurrent phlegm, having energy, and full moon winter wisdom.

Since women were forbidden to write in Renaissance times and hardly given an academic education until the 20th century, how many formulas, discoveries, vaccines, and surgery procedures were lost because the village wise women were silenced?

Women are reclaiming women's rights, and healing is still a woman's rite. This is a heroine's journey, sorting through the labyrinth of mixed messages, staid medical dictionaries, pill vs. herb charts at cross-purposes, and neoteric-plastic-fantastic-styrofoamed illnesses smothered by a badly patched Western culture reeling from the definitions of the new normal. Confluxes of online maiden-wise women brew teas and make tattoo salves while crone power recalls arcane herbalism buried deep in old-growth forests, ready to be unearthed.

> *"The history of men's opposition to women's emancipation is more interesting perhaps than the story of that emancipation itself."*
>
> *— Virginia Wolff*
>
> *With a nod to Ms. Wolff:* The history of the suppression of women's herbal healing remedies is more interesting perhaps than the story of the emancipation of that information itself.

In our modern society, women's healing circles are being reborn. Women are coming together at yoga centers, metaphysical retreats, ex-urban institutes, in groves, and in their homes. Stories and fine teas are served.

Women still die in childbirth, children are still born with birth defects, and men still need recovery from the brute force of wars. Nurturing has a long history, and allopathic medical practices have not eradicated every foible, deficiency, nor transgression. The traditional healing arts are regenerating their place again, free of harassment by uninformed physicians. There are separate narratives here about valuing the enormous clinical body of plant work left to us by Western herbalists (2,500 years old), Traditional Chinese Medicine (3,500 years old), and the traditional medicine of India, Ayurveda (5,000 years old). So how does Western medicine compete with, integrate with, and continue making money while acknowledging the existence of botanical remedies?

There is overwhelming empirical and global scientific evidence that nature's garden helps us stay healthy. The questions are: what information is needed about how the body works? How does one know which herbs to take?

Up against all these toxins and diseases, we still have our livers, kidneys, immune system, lymphatic system, and digestive system. Our bodies have an innate wisdom that recognizes pathogens and maladies. The next question is, what do today's health problems look like?

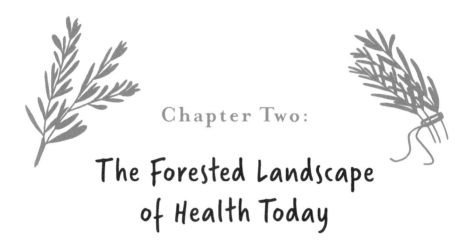

Chapter Two:
The Forested Landscape of Health Today

When Mother Nature planted her pharmacopoeia after the last ice age about 2.6 billion years ago, she foresaw health issues about forest life with plants and animals, and survival belonging to the fittest. Getting colds, eating injurious mushrooms, warrior wounds, snakebites, easing childbirth, and sustaining nourishment throughout the seasons were on her inventory of maladies. She didn't calculate as far as the 21st century and what shenanigans humankind would get into. Today, there's no scurvy because fruits aren't in season; nor food poisoning from unrefrigerated, putrid meat; nor believing a loved one was slain by a wicked demon instead of an errant, inherited gene expressing itself.

Today, it's about—

- A 35-year-old, healthy, American man spending two weeks in Australia, diving off its enormous coastline. Eight hours after his last dive, he boarded a plane for his 16-hour flight home to

> *If you don't make time for your wellness, you will be forced to make time for your illness.*
>
> — Joyce Sunada

Washington State. While in-flight, he died. Known as decompression illness, the human body was not designed to go from the depths of the ocean to 40,000 feet in the air within such a short period of time.

- Some people sit at desks all day (not bending, stooping, running, nor carrying) and stare into blue light from computers, which has led to macular degeneration, a sluggish thyroid, over-taxed adrenal glands, too much caffeine, and restless leg syndrome.

- Carpal tunnel syndrome is caused by pressure on the median nerve. Considered the most compressive neuropathy, the carpal tunnel is a narrow passageway surrounded by bones and ligaments on the palm side of your hand. When the median nerve is compressed, the symptoms can include numbness, tingling, and weakness in the hand and arm. If a person repeats the same action daily for 8 to 10 hours (assembly line, typing on a computer, etc.), this becomes a problem. It affects three to six percent of our population. (National Library of Medicine)

- Autism from too many vaccines. While much of the information linking the rise in autism to the rise in vaccines has been taken down from the internet, the statistics do show a rise in the number of autism cases concurrently with the rise of the childhood vaccinations. https://www.uofmhealth.org/health-library/ ue4907 Robert Kennedy, Jr. wrote a brilliant article about this.

- Recovery from cancer treatments. The idea of chemotherapy is to inject a "mild poison" that kills off quickly-replicating cancer cells. Along with killing off unwanted cells, it kills off healthy cells. Some side effects of chemotherapy include vomiting, brain fog, hair loss, anxiety, depression, hot flashes and menopause, weak heart, low blood cell count, digestive distress, decreased urination, cracked nails, loss of appetite, red urine, bone loss, sexual dysfunction, skin sensitivity, poor circulation, and swollen hands and feet, to name a few. https://www.healthline.com/health/cancer/effects-on-body

- Steve Belcher/weight loss product/ephedra. Ma Huang is an old and esteemed herb in Traditional Chinese Medicine. Used for respiratory health, it was brewed for the seasonal sneezing of hay fever. Scientists isolated an extract from Ma Huang called ephedrine, a chemical that acts to speed up a body's energy levels. In a misguided use of this extract, ephedrine was added to some weight loss products, and too many capsules were taken in order to lose weight faster. In 2003, Baltimore Orioles player Steve Belcher went to spring training in Ft. Lauderdale, Florida where he was told to lose weight. With his professional contract hanging over his head, he began using an ephedrine-containing weight loss product, was outside in 108-degree sun, and was vigorously training athletically for too long. The 23-year-old died.

- Some breast implants made of silicone gel have leaked inside women's bodies. The symptoms have included depression, brain fog, dry mouth and dry eyes, gastrointestinal problems, rashes and skin issues, and more.

- Currently, the annual sales of medications for ADD/ADHD in the United States alone were estimated to be $17 billion annually in 2023. (ReportsandData.com) As one of the top categories of psychopharmaceutical drugs, it would seem that this health issue, *attention deficit disorder*, would be front and center in scientific global research. Not so. Cultures based on high achievement, like Israel, China, and Saudi Arabia, are revving up their purchasing of pills to press junior's focus into submission, yet the real story lies in the fact that statistics about *other countries'* spending on ADD drugs are *not to be found.* While the Centers for Disease Control can tell you state-by-state the percentage of children who've been told they need medicating, finding a list/chart/table on how often *other countries* diagnose and spend on ADD is like looking for that proverbial needle in an organic haystack. How is it that "ADD/ADHD" is overwhelming the resources of American school systems, as well as boosting the sales of prescription drugs, and *other countries are not hyperventilating* about it? Other countries are not drugging their kids, and they are finding places/jobs/roles for their children within their cultures.

- Drug abuse treatment costs the United States over $600 billion annually. (Drugabuse.gov) While marijuana has been ostracized for being a gateway drug to harder street drugs, it has been overlooked and underreported that some real gateway drugs for children and adolescents are these ADD/ADHD drugs. A number of my college students have told me how much fun it is getting a younger siblings' Adderall XR (amphetamine), Dexedrine (amphetamine), or Ritalin (Methylphenidate), and party all night, away at school, far from their parents' watchful eyes. The ADD/ADHD prescription is a steady supply source, and the younger sib gains entrepreneurial business skills when s/he starts peddling pills to the older sib's college friends. After college, many of these students graduate into designer street drugs combined with alcohol. It's hard to calculate what the effects on childhood, young adulthood, childbearing years, and senior time will be for people who've been putting synthetic substances into their bodies since adolescence.

- Heart disease and stress from crowded living conditions, office politics, keeping up with the Joneses, narcissistic/abusive relationships, and constrictive, cultural values—When Mother

Nature gave us the "fight-or-flight response," it was intended for use when a bear or an angry marauding tribe chased us through the bush. Today, psychologists and sociologists tell us that "fight or flight" kicks in when living under emotionally trying situations. Our tribal ancestors didn't face these situations, yet our bodies will go on hyperdrive, pumping adrenaline and tying knots in our intestinal tracts. The gut–brain connection is very powerful and the current subject of cartloads of studies.

- Healthy eating is a subject addressed from elementary school all the way through high school. Yet, for fundraisers, school children are directed to sell cute chocolate bars and cookies with additives and double sugar doses. High schools are anchored with soda machines.

- Curbing one's sweet tooth can be an uphill, Herculean task, especially if one has failed before. Statistics and storylines abound about the rise of both Type 1 and Type 2 Diabetes. Diabetes occurs when the body either does not make enough insulin or cannot use it effectively. Type 2 Diabetes is the gateway to more serious complications, as the excess blood sugar (hyperglycemia) results in progressive damage to large and small blood vessels. The resulting common and debilitating complications include heart disease, stroke, and the "BAD Complications" (Blindness, Amputations of lower extremities, and Dialysis due to kidney failure). Diabetes is responsible for about half of all new U.S. cases of BAD complications. The economic burden of diabetes and pre-diabetes is huge: an estimated *$322 billion.*" https://nwhn.org/the-great-diabetes-epidemic/

- Sugar was the first foodstuff to be manufactured en masse and sold to the public. Since the 1850s, the industrial revolution has supplied refined sugar for consumers in quantities the human body was never designed to handle, and statistics on Type 2 diabetes have only been increasing. In 1958, about a million and a half of Americans had type 2 diabetes; in 2023, the CDC tells us, "More than 37 million Americans have diabetes (about 1 in 10), and approximately 90–95% of them have type 2 diabetes." https://www.mayoclinic.org/diseases-conditions/type-2-diabetes/symptoms-causes/syc-20351193 https://www.cdc.gov/diabetes/statistics/slides/long_term_trends.pdf

Today, sugar is in tomato sauces for pasta, delicatessen whitefish salad, glazed pecans in salads, cling peaches, frozen turkey dinners, all those mocha-latte-whoopee frapes sold by smiling baristas, chocolate bars *and* granola bars, steak sauces, deli casseroles, fast food salads, and several hundred other unsuspecting food choices shoppers make.

Sugar (and Other Sweeteners): The Patisserie of American Cuisine

Around the fifth century BC, the famous Indian surgeon Sushruta, in his work *Samhita*, identified diabetes by using the term madhumeha (honey-like urine) and pointed out not only the sweet taste of the urine but also its sticky feeling to the touch and its ability to attract ants! Sushruta further mentions that diabetes affects primarily the rich castes and is related to the excessive food consumption as rice, cereals and sweets. (National Library of Medicine https://www.ncbi.nlm.nih.gov/pmc/articles/PMC4707300/)

Sugar occurs very infrequently in nature. Oranges, apples, bananas, mangoes, kiwi, grapes, raspberries, blueberries, and other wonderful fruits are all seasonal. When our cave mothers were picking their way through bushes, brush, and long trailing vines, they were competing with other animals in the forest, whether raccoons, bears, monkeys, or giraffes with big, long necks who picked fruit off of tree tops. By the time the keeper of the hearth got to her local apple tree, three-quarters of it had already been plucked and eaten. Whatever she finally gathered was brought back to the cave and shared. People didn't get that much sugar. Europeans introduced sugarcane to the New World in the 1490s. It then became a major cash crop between 1710 and 1770, equaling 20% of all European imports. As sugar became an industrialized, profitable product, diabetes in America rose. Recipes for baked goods "with a loaf of sugar added" were mushrooming in every goodwife's cookbook. Mason Jars were introduced in the mid-1800s, and more foods got more sugar when canned. During World War I, the British sent chocolate bars to their soldiers to boost morale and energy. After an Army Quartermaster Corps decree in December 1918, the military began issuing a half-pound of candy every 10 days to soldiers serving overseas. (Washington Post) When the soldiers came home with a sweet tooth, candy companies began to grow. When World War II happened, chocolate bars were packaged to withstand teargas (https://www.dvidshub.net) WW II veterans begat the Baby Boomers, and everyone wanted some peace, quiet, and a lollipop at the end of the day. Within the last 75 years, commercially packaged "instant" food products have been developed, and sweeteners of all kinds are added in. (See list in excipients.)

As the American marketplace has become accustomed to this heightened sweetness, statistics tell us:

- In 1647, the Portuguese found that the climate of Brazil was perfect for growing that Southeastern Asian crop, sugar. They introduced sugar to the Caribbean, and European cuisine embraced sweetened flavors at full speed ahead.

- In 1700, the average American ate four pounds of sugar per year.

- In 1800, the average American ate 18 pounds of sugar per year.

- In 1900, the average American ate 40 pounds of sugar per year.

- In 2009, the average American ate nearly 80 pounds of sugar per year.

- Today, the average American eats 17 teaspoons of sugar per day. (CDC)

- *Diabetes has risen exponentially in the past 100 years.*

- In the 1920s, 0.05% to 2% of American had diabetes.

- Today, 100 million Americans have diabetes or are pre-diabetic. (CDC)

- The more education you have, the less chance you will become a diabetic.

- The healthier and more natural your diet is, the less chance you will become a diabetic. (CDC)

High-Fructose Corn Syrup

Fructose is found in fruits, honey, and even some vegetables, including corn. Currently, up to 92% of U.S. corn is genetically engineered, in turn making its high-fructose corn syrup genetically modified. (centerforfood-safety.org) The data on genetically engineered foods states that the human body receives less nutrition and has greater, long-term health issues. Extracts of genetically engineered foods rank just as high as determents to your health. The corporate concerns' marketing machines have managed to convince the public that if a packaged food contains an artificially manufactured sweetener, but does not contain *sugar, it's better*. Artificial extracts boast about being sweeter than sugar at the same time being no-calorie. On a single day, someone could have HFCS in breakfast cereal, diet sodas, energy drinks, energy bars, pasta sauce, variety pack trays, beef and mashed potato microwave trays, pasta mac and cheese trays, or frozen, chicken enchiladas. When added together, that aggregated amount of HFCS has the potential for health risks. "Most starchy carbs, such as rice, are broken down into glucose, the basic form of carbs. However, table sugar and HFCS comprise around 50% glucose and 50% fructose.

Glucose is easily transported and utilized by every cell in your body. It's also the predominant fuel source for high-intensity exercise and various processes. In contrast, the fructose from high-fructose corn syrup or table sugar needs to be converted into glucose, glycogen (stored carbs), or fat by the liver before it can be used as fuel. Like regular table sugar, HFCS is a rich source of fructose. In the past few decades, the intake of fructose and HFCS has increased significantly." (healthlinenutrition.com)

- High intake of fructose leads to a fatty liver.

- Other research shows that the HFCS leads to liver disease faster than glucose.

- Long -term use can lead to type 2 diabetes.

- Long-term studies indicate that excessive intake of sugar, including HFCS, plays a key role in the development of obesity.

- In one study, healthy adults drank beverages containing either glucose or fructose. The two groups were compared, and the fructose drink didn't stimulate regions of the brain that control appetite to the same extent as the glucose drink.

- HFCS and sugar can lead to inflammation and heart disease.

- HFCS has no nutrient content, and the more you consume, the less room you have for nutrient-dense foods. (healthlinenutrition.com)

Aspartame

Touted as a safe, supermarket sweetener, aspartame is found in table-top sweeteners (little packets), beverages, drink mixes, sugar-free gums, candies, cereals, toothpaste, and medications. The World Health Organization has reported that aspartame is possibly a carcinogen. (If an average person drinks "over 9 cans of diet soda or the equivalent in foodstuffs per day, then it's time to worry," said the doctor spokesperson.) But who is "the average person?" If a plate falls, is glued back together, and is then tossed around, it's more likely to break again, only this time, into more pieces. Likewise, with a compromised immune system, a dysbiotic intestinal tract, and an unhealthy diet, it's unwise to ingest a substance shown to tip the scale toward contrary health. The WHO news report only said people "need to be mindful" rather than "stop consuming it." Yet other studies have shown the ill effects from aspartame for years: The National Soft Drink Association (NSDA), representing American soda makers, emphatically objected to any government approval of the deadly chemical with an extensive, detailed written testimony, including these statements: "Aspartame is inherently, markedly and uniquely unstable in aqueous media. In a liquid, such as a soft drink, APM will degrade as a function of temperature and pH. Higher temperatures and more acidic liquids increase the rate of degradation...The inability to account for as much as 39% of AMP decomposition products is significant. With such a high unknown factor, judgments about the safety of APM in soft drinks cannot be made confidently." (1983, 1985; http://www.gene.ch/gentech/1998/May-Jul/msg00127.html)

Aspartame's Metabolic Offspring

What were these unnamed "decomposition products" referred to in the NSDA's objection?

- Methyl alcohol: Class-A carcinogen, cumulative poison, narcotic. One ounce is fatal.
- Formaldehyde: Embalming fluid, kills all living things.
- Formic acid: Fire-ant poison, toxic even in minute quantities.

Aspartame contains two synthetic amino acids that are toxic when isolated. Aspartic acid (40% of APM), like MSG, is an excitotoxin. It can excite neurons to fire at an accelerated rate until they exhaust and die, and it destroys brain cells. Phenylalanine (50% of APM), is deadly, lowering the seizure threshold and depleting serotonin, triggering psychiatric and behavioral problems. Extremely harmful to the unborn, phenylalanine is neurotoxic, causing abortions, birth defects, and mental deficiency, as well as manifold neurological damage. (https://thenhf.com/curtain-fall-on-the-aspartame-follies/)

Key Facts About Aspartame

Dozens of studies have linked the popular artificial sweetener to serious health problems, including cancer, cardiovascular disease, Alzheimer's disease, seizures, stroke and dementia, as well as negative effects such as intestinal dysbiosis, mood disorders, headaches, and migraines.

Evidence also links aspartame to weight gain, increased appetite, and obesity-related diseases. (https://usrtk.org/sweetners/aspartame_health_risks)

It would be irresponsible to not recognize that the fate of this additive is attached to the financial corporate goals of aspartame. If I was teaching an economics class, this would be a fascinating discussion: scientific and empiric evidence versus a bottom line. So much of what is reported today about medicine and food chains is wrapped up in this very discussion. When choosing what to put into your body, learn both sides of the story, and then decide. Compound that unwieldy, subterranean assault on the pancreas, liver, and kidneys with the 80,000 toxins, chemicals, and preservatives we are exposed to daily, and our Garden-of-Eden bodies just cannot keep up with the digesting, processing, storing, and cleansing we ask them to do.

Weight loss is a hot-button, third-rail, first-world health issue. Adam, Eve, and the cavepeople were too busy hunting and gathering to gain weight. But today, there's every opportunity to eat processed, excipient-laden, and fattening fast foods, which quickly add pounds on. (If you haven't seen the movie, "Supersize Me" by Morgan Spurlock, I highly recommend it.) People try these stressful, strained, restrictive diets, lose some weight, return to their old habits, and regain what they lost. Clearly, something is wrong with this dieting model. The answer is two-fold: People need a good education about which foods are healthy, and they need to adjust their lifestyles for support when transiting into a healthier lifestyle. (See step 1 ½, The Buying Committee.)

Intent on eliminating economic competition, the medical–industrial complex set its sights on the resurgence of herbalism sprouting up in the 1960s.

Dietary Supplement Health and Education Act of 1994 Public Law 103-417 (DSHEA)

In the late 1960s, a scattering of botanical stores had survived in large cities where free-thinkers, eccentric intellectuals, and ethnic nomads still managed to find medicinal herbs for their needs. Then the hippies went back to the land and wanted free schools for education, blue jeans and love beads for wear, organic vegetables for food, and Mother Nature's pharmacopeia for medicine. As they matured into adulthood, started families, and experienced first-hand the cost of health insurance, they intensified their search for whole foods and nature's bounty. Supplement brands gained legitimacy, and books describing sustainable, green choices emerged touting the benefits of vegetarianism and brewing medicinal teas. The people's voices were heard. The Baby Boom generation wanted *alternative choices*. Then, in the early 1990s, Big Pharma noticed the health food industry was topping $20 billion dollars a year, and so it posed a question to Congress: How were vitamins and herbs to be regulated? As foods? As drugs? Thoughtfully, Congress came up with a very sensible solution: a third category, dietary supplements. Below are direct quotes from the law, DSHEA, to illustrate what the Federal government enacted as the major law that governs the dietary supplement industry.

DSHEA

"§2. Findings-

Congress finds that:

- (1) improving the health status of United States citizens ranks at the top of the national priorities of the Federal Government;

- (2) the importance of nutrition and the benefits of dietary supplements to health promotion and disease prevention have been documented increasingly in scientific studies;

- (3)(A) there is a link between the ingestion of certain nutrients or dietary supplements and the prevention of chronic diseases such as cancer, heart disease, and osteoporosis; and

- (B) clinical research has shown that several chronic diseases can be prevented simply with a healthful diet, such as a diet that is low in fat, saturated fat, cholesterol, and sodium, with a high proportion of plant-based foods;

- (4) healthful diets may mitigate the need for expensive medical procedures, such as coronary bypass surgery or angioplasty;

- (5) preventive health measures, including education, good nutrition, and appropriate use of safe nutritional supplements will limit the incidence of chronic diseases, and reduce long-term health care expenditures;

- (6)(A) promotion of good health and healthy lifestyles improves and extends lives while reducing health care expenditures; and

- (B) reduction in health care expenditures is of paramount importance to the future of the country and the economic well-being of the country;

- (7) there is a growing need for emphasis on the dissemination of information linking nutrition and long-term good health;

- (8) consumers should be empowered to make choices about preventive health care programs based on data from scientific studies of health benefits related to particular dietary supplements;

- (9) national surveys have revealed that almost 50 percent of the 260,000,000 Americans regularly consume dietary supplements of vitamins, minerals, or herbs as a means of improving their nutrition;

- (10) studies indicate that consumers are placing increased reliance on the use of nontraditional health care providers to avoid the excessive costs of traditional medical services and to obtain more holistic consideration of their needs;

- (11) the United States will spend over $1,000,000,000,000 on health care in 1994, which is about 12 percent of the Gross National Product of the United States, and this amount and percentage will continue to increase unless significant efforts are undertaken to reverse the increase;

- (12)(A) the nutritional supplement industry is an integral part of the economy of the United States;

- (B) the industry consistently projects a positive trade balance; and

- (C) the estimated 600 dietary supplement manufacturers in the United States produce approximately 4,000 products, with total annual sales of such products alone reaching at least $4,000,000,000;

- (13) although the Federal Government should take swift action against products that are unsafe or adulterated, the Federal Government should not take any actions to impose unreasonable regulatory barriers limiting or slowing the flow of safe products and accurate information to consumers;

- (14) dietary supplements are safe within a broad range of intake, and safety problems with the supplements are relatively rare; and

- (15)(A) legislative action that protects the right of access of consumers to safe dietary supplements is necessary in order to promote wellness; and

- (B) a rational Federal framework must be established to supersede the current ad hoc, patchwork regulatory policy on dietary supplements.

§3. Definitions

- **(a) Definition of Certain Foods as Dietary Supplements.** Section 201 (21 U.S.C. 321) is amended by adding at the end the following:

- "(ff) The term "dietary supplement"

- "(1) means a product (other than tobacco) intended to supplement the diet that bears or contains one or more of the following dietary ingredients:

- "(A) a vitamin;

- "(B) a mineral;

- "(C) an herb or other botanical;

- "(D) an amino acid;

- "(E) a dietary substance for use by man to supplement the diet by increasing the total dietary intake; or

- "(F) a concentrate, metabolite, constituent, extract, or combination of any ingredient described in clause (A), (B), (C), (D), or (E)." (https://ods.od.nih.gov/About/DSHEA_Wording.aspx)

This law validates herbal and supplement consumer choices, and protects consumers from faulty products being peddled. While a few 21st-century snake-oil salesmen have tried some lame, get-rich-quick potions and pills, what has developed since the onset of DSHEA is an industry of enormous integrity, heck-bent on self-regulation, and in a state of perpetual education and information overload. Going to the trade shows is limitless—talk, talk, talk from ancient herbology to the latest scientific studies. There are devoted followers, with supporters, pioneers, advocates, and teachers bringing the land back.

Ironically, after Congress passed DSHEA, the supplement industry exploded with its new-found legitimacy leading the way. Then the recycled hippies who'd championed alternative health had an unannounced guest: Big Pharma wanted to move back-to-the-land too. Big Pharma started buying up supplement brands and Wall Street partnerships were ready to invest in (perceived) quick-fix schemes. Instead of the slow-and-steady recovery plant medicine traditionally delivered, it was thought that executing monetized formulas for a ready-made market would be a sure-fire sale. The rhythms of nature got shelved as chemical formulators played with a new set of ingredients, looking to make a deal and call it a day. (Note: Big Pharma was also looking for another way to eliminate competition.) Currently in the marketplace there is an authoritative dance between burgeoning financial concerns and the raw-foods-sacred-cycle-mindful-plant-based partisans. Each claims ownership of the health food industry model, but it's good to remember the caveat, "Buyer beware." The solution is to learn as much as you can about your diet and nutraceuticals, and then make your choices.

A Pressing Issue: Hidden Excipients. What Are Excipients?

As DSHEA's passage by Congress quelled doubts about the efficacy of herbs, it also baited a manufacturing boom, in turn leading to other,

Of far greater potential danger to the consumer's health are the hidden contaminants and bacteria like salmonella and residues from the use of pesticides, nitrates, nitrites, hormones, antibiotics, and other chemicals. *New York Times,* July 18, 1971 (Prescription for Dietary Wellness, Balch & Balch, 1992)

unexpected events. Namely, how quickly could alternate delivery systems deliver the long-held benefits of herbs and nutrients without having to wait for the body's own metabolism to work? **Enter excipients.**

Dietary supplements, the enhanced nutritional products developed by emerging health food industry formulators to increase the transfer of nutritive constituents, come in a variety of forms, including tablets, capsules, gummies, and powders, as well as blended drinks and energy bars. Excipients are additional ingredients mixed into nutritional products (they are in both "regular" foods and "natural" foods) to disencumber the manufacturing process, assist in product identification, legitimize a trademarked product, and act as a carrier or component for the main ingredient(s). Excipients correspond to *food additives,* added ingredients for improving taste, texture, appearance, nutritional value, preservation, easing digestion, facilitating the digestive process, binding ingredients together, helping the formula move easily through the manufacturing equipment, decreasing friction between particles of the blend, and other uses in manufacturing. Excipients may be used to enhance the finished product's appearance, stability, consumer acceptance (satisfaction), and bioavailability (proportion of the active ingredient that is absorbed and available for use). Protecting, supporting, and enhancing stability improves overall safety and function of the product during transport, storage, and use. Many excipient ingredients are used for more than one function or purpose. (https://fullscript.com/blog/excipients)

Excipients in supplements are used for various functions, which include:

- Acidifying/alkalizing agent
- Aerosol propellant
- Antifoaming agent
- Antioxidant
- Binding agent
- Buffering agent
- Carrier/vehicle
- Chelating/sequestering agent
- Coating agent
- Coloring, flavor, perfume
- Diluting/bulking agent (to quantify dose accuracy)
- Disintegrant (to aid dissolution in the gastrointestinal tract)
- Emulsifier
- Filler
- Flavor agent
- Flow agent
- Glidant/anticaking agent
- Granulating agent
- Humectant (to preserve moisture)
- Lubricant
- Ointment/suppository base
- Plasticizer
- Preservative
- Stiffening agent
- Suspending agent
- Sweetener
- Thickening agent

Under DSHEA, the FDA designated specific guidelines for written labels on nutraceutical products. Ingredients are listed from the highest portion to the lowest portion. While many additives are listed, they *do not all have to be listed*. When the quantity of an additive (excipient) exceeds the allowed percentage of the finished product, the additive must be listed (these percentages vary from one ingredient to another). If the quantity of the additive (excipient) *does not exceed* the allowed percentage of the finished product, the additive (excipient) does not have to be listed. Therefore, if you are taking a number of nutraceutical products (and/or other manufactured foods), you might be exceeding an acceptable threshold of a particular additive (excipient) *in toto*. If you have an unfavorable reaction, and you won't be able to pinpoint what disrupted your homeostasis.

And then, in addition to the chemical and toxic overload, the subliminal and subconscious cues from a society loaded with violent images on social media platforms and explosive Hollywood blockbusters, coupled with volatile public conversations and familial, negative verbal patterns, puts us into the fight-or-flight mode daily. The day is also dysregulated by mechanized transportation (car accidents, motorcycle casualties, train wrecks, etc.), and dancing-as-fast-as-you-can-job stress. Modern life exhausts a mind that hardly gets a moment of rest, let alone time to smell the virtual flowers. Nature's original intention was for people to work in fields, rise with the sun and sleep with the dark, and be surrounded by a constant community of family with dependable values; there was a harmony and equilibrium

When using the herb plant itself, you'll know what you're putting into your body. When an herb is taken one-at-a-time, you will accurately be able to access your body's reaction to it. There are also established, trusted brands in a health food store which use natural preservatives and easy processes thereby eliminating the need for excessive additives.

throughout the day. Sociological studies on the effects of contemporary stress levels all point out the need for the growing businesses of yoga classes, anti-stress meds, silent retreats, one-minute meditations, in-house therapists for large corporations, elementary school social workers, and, unfortunately, the continued spread of street drugs. Every church, synagogue, temple, and mosque once served as an oasis for compartmentalized, civilized culture, yet religious institutions have been losing followers to these more immediate solutions.

The average American is now up against substance abuse, empty calories from candies and sweets, working indoors all day with little sunshine or fresh air, drugs "to limit" the number of periods a woman gets a year, severe emotional dumping by friends (in the absence of a religious refuge and nearby extended family members), PTSD, mass shootings, culture clashes, an antagonized vagus nerve, and compounding digestive issues. Most Westerners have not been educated about handling this stressful, metropolitan life, and television shows and films abound starring characters who finally "crack."

None of the fables, fairytales, and morality plays passed down by our storytellers, poets, and actors ever acquaint the modern world with how previous lineages coped with overload; their social structures were fixed in place, caretaking the daily dose of a strident life.

That Western-Medicine Mindset

There have been enormous, prodigious, and life-changing discoveries in Western medicine that have benefitted humankind: antibiotics, x-rays, ultrasounds, the appropriate use of pain medication, germ theory, blood analysis, documenting body systems, insulin, setting casts, neonatal care, and dentistry, to name a few. It is safe to say that many of us have been helped at one time or another by these.

The model of medical distribution now is also, usually, *this health issue=this particular pill.*

What television commercials, radio and print ads, television shows, Hollywood movies, bureaucratic mouthpieces, grade-school science books, brochures in doctors' offices, and paid-for online social media usually assert is that only prescribed pills correct diseases. The idea that for every malady, a doctor prescribes a drug is re-enforced again and again. This message gets delivered from all accessible socializing forces. Additionally, whereas the goodwives used to carry bundles of grain and baskets of potatoes from the fields, chatting about conditions and trading plant remedies with the other village mothers, today the message is, "You must ask the doctor." I remember watching a specific commercial about a respiratory drug, introduced during the early spring for hay fever. The last line of the commercial went, "Therefore, call this number, to get this brochure, so you can take it to your doctor, to find out if you are better." Another commercial claimed, "You'll know you're better when you go to your next check-up and see the numbers on your doctor's tests."

When I first became health conscious, the steps to handling an illness were barely written down. Where did a city dweller get herbs? Find them? Ask questions? How did you experiment? What were good results supposed to feel like? Most people don't live next to a forest for foraging. *There are other ways to gather plants and new ways to use them.*

I wanted to research how people are taught to cook, so I started watching cooking shows. Most of the shows had a gourmet touch, with lots of sugar, salt, wines, and butter added to everything. I'll admit it looked tasty. But was it healthy? One night when watching television, within the same hour, one cooking show had commercials for three of the major fast food restaurants and three of the major dieting companies. Madison Avenue labels that: strategic marketing!

Within this current renaissance of antiquarian herbalism, I am a first-generation urban herbalist. The summation here is not about scientific dissection and statistical manipulation. This book is the result of experience. I am a practicing herbalist, immersed in the daily aches, pains, cries, anguish, toil, heartaches, and disturbances from a varied collection of people from every race, walk of life, educational level, and economic status. It is my hope that the information, stories, and recipes contained herein will guide, inspire, and empower each of you.

Fast forward: My resume includes healing myself from hormonal imbalances, PTSD, migraine headaches, residual weight gain, car accidents, and leaky gut syndrome. I have taught nurses, nurse practitioners, pharmacists, and doctors, as well as newcomers to holistic health; lectured at independent health food stores as well as Whole Foods; taught herbs and nutrition at college for 12 years; contributed to a nutrition textbook for college; produced and hosted a radio show, The Urban Herbalist, for 14 years; written articles; was the regional manager for three of the major supplement brands in the health food industry; attended various trade shows and represented my companies at trade shows; done weed walks; and was the apothecary at the New York Renaissance Faire.

When you walk through the door of a health food store, you are taking back your power.

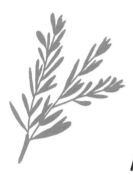

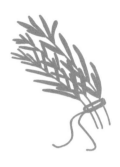

Chapter Three:

Mothercrafting Your Protocol

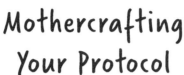

The Liver

Class motto: Love your Liver! Devoured by the biggest carnivores, the organ most affected by too much alcohol and too many drugs (legal and illegal), a transformer that conjugates foreign food cells with an endogenous molecule in order for food to be accepted in your body, and a piece of human flesh with a two-year transplant-waiting list, the liver is the largest solid organ and gland in the human body. It carries out over 400 essential tasks every day. Defining the metabolic crossroads of the body, the liver stores, packages, recycles, metabolizes, eliminates, and redistributes nutrients received from the gastrointestinal tract. It also detoxifies drugs, converts excess nitrogen to urea to be passed through the kidneys and excreted by the bladder, recycles iron, synthesizes protein, helps dismantle old red blood cells, prepares waste products for excretion, and produces chemicals for digesting food. The liver stores vitamin A, zinc, glycogen, and iron, among other nutrients. It is both a part of the digestive system and the cleansing process.

"The liver's placement ensures that it will be first to receive the nutrients absorbed from the GI tract. In fact, the liver has many jobs to do in preparing the absorbed nutrients for use by the body…The liver serves as a gatekeeper to defend against substances that might harm the heart or brain. That is why, when people ingest poisons that succeed in passing the first barrier (the intestinal cells), the liver often suffers the damage—from viruses such as hepatitis, from drugs such as barbiturates or alcohol, from toxins such as pesticide residues, and from contaminants such as mercury…The liver is the most active processing center in the body. When nutrients enter the body from the digestive tract, the liver receives them first; then it metabolizes, packages, store, or ships them out for use by other organs. When alcohol, drugs or poisons enter the body, they are also sent directly to the liver; here they are detoxified, and their by-products shipped out for excretion." (*Understanding Normal & Clinical Nutrition*)

Understanding and addressing your liver are critical to your overall health.

- Carbohydrates: makes and stores glycogen, converts fructose and galactose to glucose, breaks down glycogen and releases glucose, breaks down glucose for energy when needed, makes glucose from some amino acids and glycerols when needed, converts glucose to fatty acids.

- Proteins: manufactures nonessential amino acids that are in short supply, removes from circulation excess amino acids and coverts them to other amino acids or deaminates them to glucose or fatty acids, removes ammonia from the blood and converts it to urea for excretion, makes other nitrogen-containing compounds the body needs (such as bases used in DNA and RNA), makes plasma proteins such as clotting factors.

- Lipids: builds and breaks down triglycerides, phospholipids, and cholesterol as needed, breaks down fatty acids for energy when needed, packages extra lipids in lipoproteins, for transport to other body organs, manufactures bile for the gallbladder for use in fat digestion, makes ketone bodies when necessary.

The consequences of a damaged or diseased liver can be fatal. And a long, painful decline of a compromised liver can result in lethargy, pain, dizziness, heart issues, malnourishment, wasting, general debilitation, jaundice, edema, cardia cirrhosis, clotting abnormalities, elevated blood ammonia levels, hepatic encephalopathy, and hepatic coma with hepatitis, cirrhosis, or other illnesses.

These multiple actions and overlayered pathways of the liver are critical to understanding how your body pathways and what *receiving* nutrition versus *utilizing* nutrition really looks like. You don't just drink a class of orange juice, and the body is suddenly loaded with vitamin C, keeping the immune system on guard and slaying pathogens. An intricate digestive process has evolved over thousands of millennia to insure our growth and good health, and the allopathic-synthetic-medicine-fast-foods-diet-and-polluted lifestyle does not support this process.

There's another debate, struggle, and enigma here. The liver is an integral part of our body's health, and how did the Standard American Diet (SAD) stray so far away from nurturing it? What can we do today to make our livers well?

Our bodies still follow the rhythms and cycles of our cave-people ancestors. Our bodies were not designed for one, humongous dollop of 5,000 milligrams of vitamin C, so now we are "healthy." There is no fruit nor vegetable anywhere that has 5,000 milligrams of vitamin C, yet those horse-pills are for sale over-the-counter. This overdose of nutrients is a cousin of a belief born out Western medicine's frame of reference. Pill-pushing concerns developed mid-19th century and really gained momentum in the 1930s, when investors took their money out of the schools of homeopathy and invested in manufacturing. The big investors, Carnegie and Rockefeller, et al., knew they needed original marketing angles to capture the attention of a population weaned on herbal remedies and self-sufficient home care. A drug with the thrust to override corporeal body's rhythms and seasonal timelines was marketable; the side effects were yet to be determined.

Our bodies were designed to store, recycle, rotate, absorb, and reuse the nutrients we assimilate, not the toxins. And our livers can't keep up with what are asking them to do today.

Unprocessed toxins express themselves as headaches, fatigue, lethargy, dizziness joint pains, stomach ache, intestinal cramps coughing, wheezing, sore throat, fever, runny nose, circulation deficiencies, excessive blood fats, skin rashes, hives, frequent colds, itchy nose, irritated eyes, tearing, nausea, indigestion, bad breath, smelly feet, and diarrhea. (Haas)

Problems related to toxicity and stagnation: acne, boils, eczema allergies, breathing issues, arthritis, headaches, migraines, constipation, ulcerative colitis, hemorrhoids, diverticulitis, irritable bowel syndrome, gastritis, gout, obesity, kidney stones, uterine fibroid tumors, hepatitis, prostate disease, menstrual irregularities, diabetes, blood sugar issues, hyperactivity, mental problems, Alzheimer's disease, senility, Parkinson's disease, drug addiction, infections by bacteria, viruses, fungus, parasites, worms. (Haas)

Toxins are of much greater concern to humankind today than when Mother Nature was sitting in the Garden of Eden 200,000 years ago, sipping tea, and designing our bodies. She didn't calculate for the modern stresses and strains, physically and emotionally, nor the denatured, chemically loaded, artificial foods eaten today, as well as the chemical drugs and invasive procedures. Environmental toxins, pesticides, herbicides, industrial chemicals, radiation, nuclear power, computer blue light, and street drugs were not in her glossary of illnesses. Congested metropolis stressors, negative spiritual influences, disaffirming thought patterns, and harmful emotions also impose on our well-being. Our bio-clocks are still set to the TCM rhythms of the day, and Mother Nature devotes nearly half of our diurnal cycle to detoxification. Even back then she knew we would need renewal from our daily, natural world. There are still people living close to nature and anthropological studies along with the United Nations' research indicate their health is less fractious and incapacitating. People are in greater need of depuration more than ever.

The Biorhythm Cycles of the Meridians (Traditional Chinese Medicine)

7–9:00 a.m. stomach	7–9:00 p.m. heart constrictor*
9–11:00 a.m. spleen-pancreas	9–11:00 p.m. triple heater**
11:00 a.m.–1:00 p.m. heart	11:00 p.m.–1:00 a.m. gallbladder
1–3:00 p.m. small intestine	1:00 a.m.–3:00 a.m. liver
3–5:00 p.m. bladder	3–5:00 a.m. lungs
5–7:00 p.m. kidney	5–7:00 a.m. large intestine

*Heart constrictor relates to the function of circulation and protects the heart.

**Triple heater relates to the movement of water in the body, and connects to the restorative functional activities of all organs in the upper, middle, and lower cavities of the body.

The first half of the day, the body is building up, and the second half of the day, the body is detoxifying.

We need internal cleansing to maintain homeostasis, reduce symptoms, treat diseases, clear addictions, and prevent illnesses. Many weight loss and drug recovery plans begin with a general cleansing. There's also a spiritual renewal when eliminating pathogens and decay. A cleanse can invigorate and enliven awareness; it helps to move energies from our lower centers of digestion up to our hearts, minds, and higher consciousness. *Recharging* is a necessity of a daily regimen.

When building a health protocol, work with the body's own cycles, so include detoxification later in the day. Likewise, seasonal changes affect our rhythms too. After the holiday season (the season of sugar), it's good to cleanse and recharge for the New Year. Just as resolutions are being made, out with old and in with the new works for our bodies too. After big events, like going to a wedding with rich foods or going on vacation to new country with exotic flavors, spices, and stressors associated with international travel, the body welcomes a chance to recover. Beginning a new job or a moving to a new home does affect your inner peace, so also factor in some down time and cleansing.

One more reason to detoxify: Ingesting denatured foods and chemical-laden antidotes can cause digestive issues. Your very tender intestinal tract can become encrusted with old fecal matter, thereby interfering with the body's ability to assimilate a nutrient-rich, plant-based diet. Unless your digestive system can *effectively assimilate the foods you eat*, then the foods and supplements taken can be wasted, eliminated without conveying their benefits. With all their food preservatives and artificial ingredients, Americans have the most expensive urine in the world.

Budding herbalists today face another conundrum: Which problem to address first? Are you not sleeping because your body is overloaded with expresso and energy-booster shots? Are you not sleeping because you're on six daily medications from the doctor, and when the chi of your body goes to the liver at 1:00 a.m., it's too busy self-cleansing, so you're awakened? Are you not sleeping because you ate wheat pasta with toma-toes and cheese on top which kicked up your immune system, thereby inflaming your intestinal tract? Has the stress of constant bickering with your spouse led to deep anxiety, so you can't recognize signals from your body? Did you just get another round of vaccinations? Did you just move more than 7 degrees longitude or 7 degrees latitude? Are you working in a building over 150 years old, and the mold throughout the airshafts and plumbing system haven't been cleaned for over a century?

> "There are two ways to reach truth— literature and agriculture."
>
> — Chinese proverb

Guidelines for Seasonal Resetting

When the seasons are changing, plan for five to seven days to: Drink juices including spirulina or chlorophyll powders. Have one meal daily of raw or cooked vegetables. Eat brown rice dishes with vegetables to stabilize biorhythms. Include detoxification herbs at breakfast, lunch, and dinner. Sip lemon juice in your apple juice or teas daily. Use oat bran or psyllium husks daily for colon cleansing. Saunas, steam baths, herbal wraps, facial steaming, massage, and chiropractic adjustments are good to schedule too. Daily stretching, walking, and other exercise will rev up circulation.

> If you see your skin breaking out, feel fatigued, or even "un-crave" a sugar shot, these are good signs. Your body is releasing.

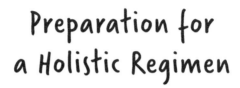

Chapter Four:

Preparation for a Holistic Regimen

Widows, goodwives, aunties, and maidens skillfully navigated between the dangers and delights of old-growth forests, coming back with armfuls of flowers and leaves for simmering into potions and teas. The keeper of the hearth was traditionally expected to be her home's healer, mothercrafting for each family member. If you want to connect to your female ancestors in your family tree, read their diaries, letters, and cookbooks for their original, foraged remedies. "I just boiled this new root for Uncle Elmo's rheumatism..." When auntie found something restorative, she quickly shared it with female family members, because illnesses traveled within families. Women were called upon to sew flesh back together torn by bear claws, pacify hysterics, rid the flesh of chicken pox, soothe an enflamed throat, banish monthly menstrual cramps, and tend a laboring mother. How did they manage? They kept "cookbooks" that were actually "cooking/healing diaries," where remedy recipes were written along with mince pies, hearty custards, and moon-phase brews. Therein, you'll unearth the deep roots in your family tree, and see how very smart great-great-great grandma really was.

> When the elderly die, a library is lost, and volumes of wisdom and knowledge are gone.
>
> —African proverb

A student asked, *which kind of migraine? From anxiety? From wind or allergies or stress or an overload of medications? From too much traveling by car, train, plane?* Shorthand tips abound on social media. This almonds-for-headaches tidbit doesn't explain how to return the body to homeostasis. Info bites are served up on a platter making them sound like replacements for the strong medications prescribed by doctors. Better to gather pieces of nutritive advice carefully as you walk the walk.

"What happens when you eat strawberries every day?" (#nature the cure/#healthytipsters) Strawberries help keep you slim, fight cancer, prevent heart attacks, increase your energy, strengthen your vision, keep your blood vessels healthy, help repair your body, lower your bad cholesterol, regulate blood sugar, and keep your brain young." Strawberries do help, but you're not taking a commercially researched, chemically-compounded medication. When a variety of fruits and vegetable are eaten together over the course of a few days, collectively, they do promote good health. The inference here is that one piece of fruit is "a pill" to heal you. The body knows what to store, mix together, and use. As your hormone messengers signal each physical and mental need, the right remedies are released from your storehouse.

Seen in a cookbook:

"Easy on the cayenne, it is very hot, but good for circulation and heart disorders." Circulation is good for the heart, but there are other ways to get there. Cayenne, which comes from a nightshade, will exacerbate inflammation, auto-immune diseases, and irritate a compromised intestinal tract. Take the good with the bad? Or, *find other tasty flavors.*

Nightshades and the off-limits List, et al.

"A legendary Washington hostess" used to be a moniker for an intelligent, ambitious woman on her way to accruing power. This vantage ground for a hostess included directing avenues of communication, not only political debate topics, but also kitchen table topics of acculturation within families. What were/are/will be the social norms? A clever hostess, Deborah, gives parties including flamboyant artists and writers, peppered with trending politicians. Excited about romping through the supermarket, she pulled me along one day for party planning. After excavating a dozen television cooking shows, she was armed with every excuse to smother her recipes in butter, sugar, salt, sour cream, whipped cream, tomatoes, red, green, and yellow peppers, and tabasco sauce. "Too much food makes for good fellows!" she chirped.

"Isn't everyone on a diet?" I tried.

"You know nobody diets on a Saturday night." She had me there. Many Western palates do crave fun foods, and when the custom becomes outdoing a rival party's fare, the edibles on a Saturday night are often the pinnacle of the no-no, off-limits food list.

One category on the off-limits list worth examining is **the night-shades**. Nightshade refers to any of several of the plants of the genus Solanum, *n., deadly. Belladonna.* (Taber's) The No No Song, sung by Ringo Starr, is a winsome reminder of the youthful, "playful substances" left behind aa we mature. Likewise, there're foods found throughout the Standard American Diet (SAD) that need leaving behind to help relieve the body of exacerbated inflammation and allergies. When a person's body is "distracted" by its autoimmune detector having to deal with nightshades, the body's vital energy, chi, is lowered. When the chi is drained, it is harder to stay well. Even though the infamous belladonna (pale deadly nightshade) is still used in homeopathy, it's a plant widely listed as poisonous because chewing even a few leaves can kill you. (Taber's) An ophthalmologist may try a solution derived from belladonna to dilate your pupils in order to examine the widened pupils of your eyes; the body's response is so extreme because the plant is so potent. "Belladonna drops act as a muscarinic antagonist, blocking receptors in the muscles of the eye that constrict pupil size." (Wikipedia) Individual compounds make a belladonna extract into a narcotic or sedative. Not all the nightshades have such dramatic effects, but multiplied together, their effects can be formidable for someone coping with an auto-immune disease. Research has found that when people with disordered immune responses stopped consuming all varieties of nightshades, their conditions improved. While there are ninety-two genera with over two-thousand species of nightshades, these are the most commonly found in the Western cuisine.

The Nightshades' Off-Limits List

- Belladonna
- Sacred datura
- Tobacco
- Brugmansia
- Petunia
- Potato
- Tomato
- Tomatillo
- Eggplant
- Naranjilla
- Bell peppers: red, orange, yellow, and green
- Paprika, chili pepper, cayenne, and curry
- Ashwaganda
- Pimento
- Goji berry (wolfberry)
- Cape Gooseberry
- Pepino

- Garden huckleberry
- Mandrake
- Henbane
- Jalapeno
- Tabasco pepper
- Tabasco sauce
- Habanero
- Carolina horsenettle
- Black nightshade (European black nightshade)
- Yellow fruit nightshade (Indian nightshade)
- Silverleaf nightshade
- Bittersweet

The Spaniards brought tomatoes, potatoes, and peppers back to Europe in the sixteenth century. Versatile ingredients and easily cultivated, they proliferated and inspired royal cuisine as soon as a king's kitchen boy could deliver seedlings to the next castle. They're still favorite ingredients, especially for cooks whose special flavor is "hot-hot-hot." Note: nightshades, even tobacco, are put into cosmetics as well as dietary supplements. Anything put *on* your body topically, goes *into* your body through the epidermis. Read labels carefully. And while I love the violet petunias in my garden, I always wear thick gardening gloves when pruning. Nightshades are staples in many cuisines, including Italian, Hispanic, African-American, French, health food store deli bars, bestselling cook books, and clusters of television and podcast cooking shows. Granted, they add flavor and texture to meat, poultry, fish, and salads, yet there are other ways to spice up a recipe.

Nightshades are known to antagonize autoimmune illnesses and shown to kick up the body's immune system a notch, in turn creating inflammation, pain, migraines, bloating, constipation, diarrhea, digestive issues, fatigue, recurring fevers, swollen glands, swelling, redness, and trouble concentrating. Moreover, with tobacco on the list, it's one more reason to quit smoking.

Nightshades contain alkaloids, chemicals products of plant metabolism with a strong physiological effect on people. Alkaloids, like proteins, have a high nitrogen count, but are in fact "denatured proteins;" instead of being tissue builders, they are stimulants, hallucinogens, medicines, and poisons. The presence of nitrogen also makes them alkaline, so they neutralize acidity. Included in the better-known alkaloids are caffeine (in coffee, espresso, some intense green teas, and famously manufactured energy-boosting drinks). In the nightshade family are nicotine, atropine, belladonna, and scopolamine. Storage conditions that include extended heat and light may increase the solanine content to toxic levels. Improperly stored old potatoes have been known to cause gastrointestinal inflammation, nausea, diarrhea, dizziness, and other symptoms so severe that they may require hospitalization. (Childers) Studies have shown that there is a connection between these alkaloids which inhibit normal cartilage repair in the joints or promote the inflammatory degeneration of the joint. (Murry) *Originally found to be poisonous, tomatoes began as an ornamental plant.*

In other developments, cattle grazing on the nightshade solanum malacoxylon grow sick and deformed from an excess of vitamin D, which causes an increase of calcium (more than dairy) and phosphate in the blood, which can lead to calcification of the aorta, kidneys, lungs, and the back of the neck. (Davis/Childers) Among other effects is the calcification of soft tissue and deposit of calcium in inappropriate places within the body, one of the most prevalent symptoms in an industrial society. Hans Selye has called it "the calciphylactic syndrome," and it's involved in arthritis, arteriosclerosis, coronary disease, cerebral sclerosis, bone spurs, kidney stones, rheumatoid arthritis, chronic bronchitis, osteoporosis, erythematosus, hypertension, and even certain forms of cancer. Nightshades may remove calcium from the bones and deposit it into joints, kidneys, arteries, and other parts of the body. This becomes understandable when the acid–alkaline balance is considered.

How did humans start drinking animal's milk? Data confirms that Neolithic farmers in Northern Europe were likely the first to begin milking animals for human consumption. Western culture's inclusion of dairy in the diet has been traced back nearly 10,000 years to a time when nomadic tribes had just begun to settle down and farm. Yet, getting food was still a constant, daily, often desperate struggle. Affix to that the medical problems faced by isolated women in childbirth, in cold, wintry villages. According to medieval records, as many as one in three women died in childbirth, and in all likelihood, the death rate for mothers was even higher 10,000 years ago. That figure doesn't include women dying after having had four to eight births in as many years, infants dying within their first year, and children born with deformities. While our ancestors hadn't discovered vitamins, minerals, and the basic food groups, nor conquered the seasons, invented refrigeration, and stumbled upon pasteurization, they knew instinctively that a newborn needed a mother's milk. Probably, a woman was giving birth in a peasant hamlet one frosty, winter night, and the village women had gathered to give her comfort and aid. While their husbands sadly watched, the mother died during the birth, the women were holding the newborn, there was a goat, and somebody said, "Let's try the goat's milk." And it worked. Goat's milk is closer to human milk in composition than cow's milk, and in today's language, that goat's milk was organic, grass-fed, and without artificial hormones, steroids, nor pesticides. Later, as animals' milk was working for infants, the peasants realized they'd found a reliable form of food. Humans drank goat's milk, then cow's milk, and then other dairy products evolved over time. Yogurt came later, from curdled camel's milk in the desert. Survival—the kind of news that spread as fast as a yeoman's legs could carry him.

In our culture, nightshades are often paired with dairy foods: meat and potatoes, eggplant and parmigiana, stuffed peppers and mozzarella. It's a prominently promoted combination in Western cuisine. Additionally, dairy saturates the menu: butter, buttery dips, sour crème dips, crème sauces, cheese dishes, cheese cake, hyperbolized-buttered pancakes, French toast, buttermilk biscuits, and bagels with cream cheese are just the beginning. Our bodies stop producing the enzyme necessary to digest dairy after the age of four. In Mother Nature's book, we have been weaned from our mother's breast; therefore, we don't need to produce lactase for digesting dairy anymore.

Bacteria that support the intestinal tract can provide benefits. Using a plant-based yogurt can be a safer choice. Coconut milk, almond milk, cashew milk, soymilk, coconut milk yogurt, and almond milk yogurt are delicious for snacking and use in recipes. "Plant compounds can be potent neurotoxins if taken in quantity and can cause a syndrome similar to Parkinson's disease in animals such as horses. Solanum-tie steroidal alkaloids found in such plants as potatoes or the silver nightshade (Solanum eleagnifolium) that grows in the Sonoran Desert among ironwood trees are cholinesterase inhibitors affecting the nervous system. Animals ingesting large quantities (or sometimes smaller amounts from plants that produce them in more potent forms) can experience apathy, drowsiness, salivation, labored breathing, trembling, ataxia, and muscle weakness. At higher doses, such compounds can cause convulsions, paralysis, unconscious-ness, coma, and death." (Buhner) If the intestinal process is compromised (from other conditions, such as IBS, colitis, constipation, inflammation, or diverticulitis), then faulty signaling could result in too much calcium being extracted from bones with the excess being redistributed to the soft tissues as spurs, plaques, stones, or other calcification. The vitamin D3 in the solanum nightshades has been found to be involved in promoting the calcification of other body tissues. Today, vitamin D "fortified" foods are found in every supermarket—milk, milk powder, margarine, orange juice, breakfast cereals, and other packaged foods. With so much research, details, scientific evidence, as well as empiric evidence, nightshades are still regularly hailed as "healthy" for everyone. If you already have an autoimmune disease, suspect you have an autoimmune disease, have a relative with an autoimmune disease, or simply have some of the symptoms of an autoimmune disease, *why not try leaving all of the nightshades out of your diet for two months?* It cannot hurt. As your health issues dissipate, observe how you feel after this two-month abstention. Combine a nightshade-elimination diet with detoxification herbs, and experience a healthier difference in your body. People with autoimmune diseases, myself included, have reported less inflammation and distress when the nightshades were eliminated.

Some Autoimmune Diseases Are:

- Type 1 diabetes
- Multiple sclerosis
- Inflammatory bowel disease
- Ulcerative colitis
- Grave's disease
- Hashimoto's thyroiditis
- Autoimmune vasculitis
- Celiac disease
- Rheumatoid arthritis
- Pernicious anemia
- Crohn's disease
- Rh factor birth
- Myasthenia gravis
- Sjogren's syndrome
- Addison's disease
- Systemic lupus erythematosus
- Psoriasis/psoriatic arthritis

https://www.healthline.com/health/autoimmune-disorders#common-autoimmune-diseases

More for the Off-Limits List: Gut Assailants

- Processed sugar
- Artificial sweeteners
- Duplicate drugs/antibiotics
- Genetically modified foods (GMOs)
- Excessive fiber, colonics, and laxatives
- Sugar alcohols, alcohols
- Stress
- Fluoride
- Gluten
- Dairy
- Chemical hand sanitizers
- Highly processed foods
- Artificial flavoring, preservatives, and excipients

- Eliminating sodas, of any kind—diet, regular, classic, zero-calories, unsweetened, lightly sweetened, small, medium, large, international, subterranean, grande, and deluxe—can help. Soda contains a high amount of sugar, which promotes cavities, interacts with mouth bacteria, promotes diabetes and obesity, and corrupts your tastebuds. The high amount of phosphates affects calcium and bone metabolism. Caffeine in colas can agitate children and begin the process of caffeine addiction, which sets children up to become coffee drinkers. Instead, discover one of the playful, store-bought tea blends, create a tea blend on your own, or have a nice glass of juice.

- Blue Cheese. The penicillin mold that makes the blue stripe in blue cheese is the same mold that makes penicillin. If you are allergic to penicillin, it's best not to use blue cheese dressing nor crumpled blue cheese on salads or any other dish. Even with mixed data about ingesting the various strains of penicillin, given the growing problem of supply chain adulteration, coupled with the corrupted gut biomes of 85% of Americans, it seems foolhardy to eat something with so much potential for harm. "The data is inconclusive" may make you think "you-can-do-a-little." As one ages, the hypersensitivity to penicillin, as well as other allergens, increases. (The idea is to simplify the diet for fewer irritants.) Some side effects can be severe migraines, inflammation, breathing issues, rashes, hives, itchy eyes, swollen lips, tongue, or face, and adverse reactions to other future drugs. (In rare cases, an allergy to penicillin can cause an anaphylactic reaction, which can be deadly.)

- Dairy. Between the ages of four and five, the human body stops producing the enzyme necessary to digest dairy. In Mother Nature's book, humans have been weaned from their mother's breast by four, so lactase isn't needed anymore. She wants our bodies working on the building blocks of growing up, getting us to puberty, and beginning the intricate, hormonal developmental process. Dairy is defined as any product that can be traced back to a mammary gland. Cow's milk, goat's milk, camel's milk, butterfat milk, condensed milk, dried milk, crème, half & half, skimmed milk, low-fat milk, koumiss, kefir, cheeses, cottage cheese, cream cheese, sour cream, butter, and ice cream are all on the dairy list.

- Yogurt is a different kind of product since it contains acidophilus, friendly bacteria. Try plant-based yogurts. (Also, if the goal is to get calcium for building bones, dark, green leafy vegetables are loaded with calcium.)

The Grains Storehouse

Wheat has the highest gluten content. Gluten is a tough, sticky, nitrogenous substance that forms mucus and coats the villi of the intestines. If the villi get too heavily coated, nutrients cannot be absorbed, resulting in malabsorption. This also affects the myelin sheath of nerves. Gluten is not recommended for the ill. (Balch & Balch)

Grains are a basic, whole food found all over the earth. They are sources of complex carbohydrates, B vitamins, minerals, including magnesium, zinc, iron, potassium, calcium, phosphorus, and copper. One of the great differences between our ancestral diet and the industrial, Western diet of today is the amount of fiber we get from grains. Medical evidence has shown that a low-fiber diet is connected to numerous diseases, and a high-fiber diet is connected to the improvement of these diseases. The evolution of this Western diet includes increased fats, refined flour, white sugar, and chemicals. These factors contribute to symptoms and diseases such as colon cancer, possibly other cancers, constipation, hemorrhoids, diverticulitis, gallstones, gall bladder problems, high cholesterol, heart disease, ulcers, varicose veins, and various forms cognitive decline (the gut–brain connection). Having regular bowel movements is a positive step towards good health, and the regular consumption of whole grains, vegetables, and herbs is the optimum way to reach that goal. (Haas) Gluten is a complex protein, with valued "elastic" properties important to baking and food processing when folded into recipes at home and in restaurants. Yet, gluten-containing grains can adversely affect your digestive tract and other body systems. An allergy to gluten is not to be ignored; there are levels of gluten sensitivity, and a greater display of this is *celiac disease*. Briefly defined as "intestinal malabsorption characterized by diarrhea, malnutrition, bleeding tendency, and hypocalcemia," celiac disease is an immune system reaction to the protein contained in wheat, barley, and rye in the small intestine. Sometimes an inherited condition, celiac disease also results in the malabsorption of nutrients from the small intestine. This autoimmune response can start a chain-reaction to other impairments if needed nutrients are compromised. A number of components surround gluten sensitivity: Celiac disease spectrum, most notably, gliadin, glutenin, secalin proteins in rye, hordein proteins in barley, and the two amino acid building-blocks, proline and glutamine, which prevent the breakdown of gluten into small, harmless molecules. For people with celiac disease, glutamine and proline-rich fragments or peptides are toxic. Serious health problems like anemia, osteoporosis, infertility, brain fog, malnutrition, infertility, liver disease, irritable bowel syndrome, and intestinal cancer can result from untreated celiac disease. While some nutraceutical brands offer digestive enzymes for people with gluten sensitivity, it's best to eliminate all gluten from one's diet.

As science investigates the finer nuances in digestive issues between wheat allergies, celiac disease, and non-celiac gluten sensitivity, it's important to note the increasing rise of **leaky gut syndrome.** Leaky gut syndrome is when an unhealthy gut lining has large cracks or holes in the mucosal lining, which allow partially digested food, toxins, bugs, and other ingested chemicals to penetrate into body tissues. Normally, correctly digested food is properly absorbed through healthy villi where it's conducted into the body and transformed into the living body itself. When the correct process of digestive transformation does not take place, and these particles enter one's bloodstream through gut-lined holes; this signals the body that "foreign invaders" are present. The body's immune system is programmed to react, "to attack a foreign invader." This over-active immune response triggers inflammation and changes in the gut flora (normal bacteria), which can lead to problems within the digestive tract and the rest of the body. Today, the research world is flourishing with studies about the connections to intestinal bacteria, inflammation, and the development of several common chronic diseases.

Suffice it to say that the culprits for causing leaky gut can be genetics, improperly cooked foods, indigestible foods, bad bacteria, harsh drugs, artificial chemicals, additives, alcohol use, low-fiber diets, excessive enemas, laxatives, colonics, and other invasive probes. These are danger signals for autoimmune issues. Irritable bowel disease (IBS), Crohn's disease, headaches, and brain fog can all be negatively impacted by the worsening of a leaky gut.

According to the National Institute for Health, about two million people have celiac disease. Statistics vary; from 30% to 80% of Americans are affected by leaky gut syndrome. If you're uncertain whether you have leaky gut, you can be tested by a doctor. What is effective for helping a leaky gut is a strict gluten-free diet, eliminating other foods to which you are allergic, detoxification, and using herbs to help heal the intestinal lining.

Grains allowed in a gluten free diet:

- Amaranth,
- Arrowroot
- Buckwheat
- Corn
- Flax
- Legumes/beans
- Millet
- Nuts and seeds
- Quinoa
- Rice sorghum
- Soy tapioca
- Squash
- Yucca
- Wild rice

Foods to avoid:

- Couscous
- Wheat (wheat starch, wheat bran, wheat germ, cracked wheat, wheat berries, hydrolyzed wheat protein)
- Barley
- Rye
- Triticale
- Derivatives: spelt, durum, bulgar, emmer, semolina, farina, farro, graham, khorasan wheat, and einkorn

Processed foods to check for gluten-containing ingredients:

- Bouillon cubes
- Brown rice syrup
- Candy
- Cereals
- Chips
- Cold cuts, hot dogs, salami, sausage
- Communion wafers
- Granola bars
- Gravy
- Matzah or Matzo
- Oatmeal (may be processed in a factory that processes gluten-containing grains)
- Ready-made baking mixes
- Sauces
- Soups
- Soy sauce
- Frozen foods containing toppings (Life Extension)

Take advantage of 21st century supermarkets—there're many gluten-free crackers, pastas, sauces, matzah, and mixes out there waiting to be tried. Again, it can be worth it to try a gluten-free diet, even for just a few weeks; you'll learn more about your body.

The Undervalued Truth about Canola Oil

According to the mainstream media, canola oil is "heart healthy" and a good source of monounsaturated fats similar to olive oil. Too much of the mainstream media is influenced by skillful marketing. Canola oil is cheap to produce, so they try to convince you canola is a "health oil," leading to consumers, restaurants, and institutions stocking up on it as a viable choice. Here is the troublesome, undervalued truth about canola oil.

A Marketing Makeover: Finding Canola Oil

During World War II, it was all hands on deck to plant Victory Gardens, stitch patches on your pants, carpool instead of wearing out your tires, and find substitutes for basic commodities, since America needed to feed the Allied troops and embattled European nations. America was also scrambling to build machinery for the massive war effort:

- The Lionel toy train company started producing items for warships, including compasses.
- Ford Motor Company produced B-24 Liberator bombers.
- Alcoa, the aluminum company, produced airplanes.
- The Mattatuck Manufacturing Company, which had made upholstery nails, switched to making cartridge clips for Springfield rifles. (www.defense.gov/News)

A necessary accessory to accompany every kind of machinery is a lubricant, some kind of oil to keep the machinery moving. And during World War II, it had to be quick and cheap to produce.

Enter rapeseed oil.

It is thought the Romans introduced rapeseed oil to Europe, and it became quite valuable in the Middle Ages when farming was being organized into a science. The plant itself was handy as a "break crop," meaning it could be tilled back into the soil for nutrients and keeping out weeds. (www.duchessoil.co.uk) As the Industrial Revolution took over the West, a new use for rapeseed oil was found: lubricating steam engines and boats. Rapeseed oil had an unsurpassed benefit: it could stick to wet metal. Rapeseed was then reserved solely for machinery oil and occasionally fed to cattle, as it was largely unpalatable and contained a toxic substance called erucic acid. "Due to it having a high level of glucosinolate and erucic acid, it was originally produced as lubricant for oil lamps and later, for machinery. Chainsaws need oiling, to help minimize friction and resistance as the chain spins at high speed. Rapeseed oil is used straight in heated fuel systems and newer engine cars or blended with petroleum distillates for powering older cars. It's also frequently combined with fossil-fuel diesel, in rates varying from 2% to 20% biodiesel. (When) **processing rapeseed for oil, (it) produces an equally useful by-product.** Namely, a high protein animal feed, that is fed to cattle pigs and chickens. This meal is high-protein, competitive with soybean." (https://www.duchessoil.co.uk/news-articles/2016/5/14/7-unusual-facts-about-rapeseed)

During World War II, America couldn't get what it needed from its regular suppliers in Europe and Asia, ground-zero battlegrounds. Yet rapeseed oil—plentiful and available in Canada—was grown commercially with the retaliatory determination of the British Empire. Since rapeseed production was expanding, making money, and gaining power, the question became how to keep business going when the wartime effort was over.

The Canadians were able to super-induce manufacturing and originated an oil low in erucic acid and glucosinolate—the bitter substances that made rapeseed oil unpalatable—thereby making it edible for humans and cattle. (www.duchessoil.co.uk)

This commercially engineered foodstuff began to be marketed in the West in 1973 under its newly invented name, canola oil, **Can**ada **o**il **l**ow **a**cid.

"Canola" oil is simply a trademarked name for low-erucic acid, glucosinolate, rapeseed oil. Rumors claimed that **canola oil was high** in some fatty acids and was not safe for human consumption. The types of **fatty ingredients** included in the oil (glucosinolate and erucic acid) can be dangerous for the human body. Additionally, food manufacturers could not continue using polyunsaturated oils and make health claims about them in the face of growing evidence of their dangers. "Polyunsaturated fats, as well as sugars, are known to initiate or augment several diseases, such as cancer, inflammation, asthma, type 2 diabetes, atherosclerosis, and endothelial dysfunction." (Vanderbilt University) Nor could manufacturers return to using (discredited) traditional, saturated fats—butter, lard, tallow, and palm oil—without causing turmoil. (Another business consideration was that these fats cost far too much for the huge profit margins wanted by post-war industry.) Business executives managed to get canola oil placed on shelves in the natural foods section, and it's become an "all-natural" staple among the oils, even though in its natural state, rapeseed oil is not palatable for human consumption. Later, the American Heart Association would join together with industry to promote "vegetable oils." The idea presented by government agencies and departments of nutrition in universities was that polyunsaturated oils were better for the circulation—that is, the heart—since saturated fats could block arteries. However, by the late 1970s, the use of the polyunsaturated oils in canola oil had been associated with Keshan's disease, heart arrhythmia, and cardiac arrest. (As "vegetable oils" have been increasingly promoted since the late 1970s, the rates of obesity, inflammation, and autoimmune diseases have gone up in America.)

The 17-step process to extract "oil" from these non-edible seeds includes using hexane as a solvent for exacting the "oil," and then it has to be "winterized and bleached." The more industrial-factory steps there are between pulling a plant out of the ground and putting in on the table, the higher the likelihood there will be digestive-health issues. Remember, real food can simply be gathered from the forest and just eaten. According to "The Great Con-ola," (The Weston A. Price Foundation), the solution was to extol monounsaturated oils, such as olive oil. Studies had shown that olive oil has a better effect than polyunsaturated oils on cholesterol levels and other blood parameters, and *canola oil was monounsaturated.*

As the health food industry began to thrive, so did a number of crossover products, in this case, cooking oils, and food chains, both health food and suburban supermarkets, gladly took on the mantle of promoting this new addition to the cooking oil section.

It's okay to ask in a restaurant if they're cooking with canola oil (or any other ingredient unhealthy for you) and to request a substitute.

What are the best monounsaturated fats in foods and oils?

Nuts, avocado, olive oil, sunflower oil, sesame oil, peanut oil.

What are the best polyunsaturated fats in foods and oils?

Grapeseed, flaxseed, sunflower, soybean, safflower, fish oil.

Mother Nature's Native American Son

It was 1912, in Florida. "Bring the basket, Calvin," his grandfather always said when he arrived at his grandson's house. His grandfather meant the woven basket of palmetto reeds handmade by the Seminole tribe nearby. Calvin's grandfather was Creek—Seminole and would take the young boy wildcrafting through luscious acres of the Everglades. They went to weedy clearings to gather roots, leaves, and bark for healing soups and salves before the full tropical sun rose at high noon. Flowers bloomed and roots burrowed down, hiding and seeking, so gathering became a game. While Calvin's three other African American grandparents did more of the family's homesteading, he tagged gleefully after this grandfather on those apprenticeship swampland walks, listening for alligators and scouting plants at their peak. They would identify and choose, cut and dig, nibble and talk all those muggy mornings long. Later, back at the wooden clapboard house, surrounded by spartina grasses and cypress trees bedecked in Spanish moss, they chopped, sliced, and simmered their cuttings to make good root soups and healing balms for mosquito bites and other infections. Calvin, now in his 90s, would regularly visit my health food store, Herbs-on-Hudson, for chamomile and sarsaparilla. I asked him if his grandfather had taught him the herb names in Seminole. "Yes, but I've forgotten them all now. There's no one left to practice them with." We began recalling the plant names his grandfather taught him. When Calvin came to the shop thereafter, he enjoyed ordering in Seminole.

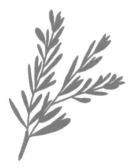

Chapter Five:

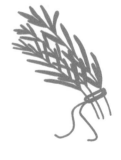

Initiation and Getting Started

How does it feel when you begin using medicinal herbs? When will you be all better?

Complete numbness to pain, relief from a headache, a purging of the intestinal tract or relief from diarrhea, cessation of coughs—the triumphs of morphine. Not to be overlooked, yet these reactions were based on the excessive potency this drug conveyed. In that specified moment of time, it *did deliver something.* One of the most significant ways pharmaceuticals beat out herbal teas in the early 20th century was by the very fact that the patient *felt something very quickly* after popping a pill. The patient was not entirely well, but the patient felt better. However, the long-term effects of taking drugs weren't in the conversation; no one recognized the internal damage to organs, nor had the addictive attributes of certain medications been observed. Perhaps people beginning an herbal protocol for rehabilitation and restoration need to ask a different question: How long will it be before my body is detoxified, restored, and feeling better?

Some people are still wired for Western, allopathic medicine and hold a vision of an uninjured, unscathed, and un-diseased body after one or two doses of a drug after a day or two of treatment. The acrobatic somersault of morphine's debut in the 1800s set the standard for using drugs. "Opium was also a major remedy for diarrhea and other diseases that spread through army camps during the Civil War. America's first opioid epidemic took shape on the battlefields of the Civil War, where physicians prescribed opium gum, laudanum, or morphine to treat the pain of gunshot wounds, and other injuries, as well as diarrhea and cough." The medicines took away pain; they worked well—too well, in fact. "Countless veterans became addicted to opium and morphine, which they continued to take after leaving the army." (Virginiahistory.org)

Morphine was sold under no restraints until 1914, when it was then classified as a "controlled substance." By the 1930s, morphine addiction was severe and use of it was spreading to other parts of the population. "It was also used for euthanasia—Sigmund Freud, being treated for inoperable jaw cancer, died from an intentional overdose of morphine administered by his physicians." (sciencedirect.com)

When an herbalist is weighing someone's health issues, the questions include:

- What are the health issues the person wants to discuss?

- How many medications is the person currently taking? Medications in the last ten years?

- How toxic is this person's body from diet, working conditions, home environment?

- How much stress is this person under?

- Does the person feel depressed?

- What is the medical history, from diseases, accidents, and inherited conditions?

- Is the person actively under the care of any physicians now? Which ones? Why?

- What surgeries has the person had? Have any organs been removed?

- Any broken bones?

- Any implants?

- Any serious childhood illnesses or adult illnesses?

- How much exercise does the person get?

- Does this person partake in alcohol, recreational drugs, or cigarettes?

- What is this person's daily schedule? A student? A mom with four kids at home? A corporate executive who flies away for business seven to ten days per month? A scientist in the South Pole conducting experiments on penguins? A stockbroker on Wall Street with a laptop on an island off the South Carolina coast? A real estate broker studying for an MBA at night?

All of this information goes into the herbalist's brainpan to be weighed, stirred, sifted, and measured. Various herbs are chosen for beginning the treatment, the middle bridge-healing, and the endgame of wellness.

Healing with herbs is not "sudden," like some headaches gone with two aspirins or a urinary tract infection ceasing with antibiotics. The body's healthy response arises slowly as the body flushes out the toxins and brightens up with nourishment. The more drugs—recreational or previous prescriptions—to be cleared out, the more stress to neutralize, the more previous broken bones and surgeries to be knitted back together, the more time the body requires to be well. And the body works on this daily. Your body wants to heal and is always reaching for it. Awakening each morning feels happier and happier.

The beginning may be waking up more refreshed, easier to focus, and a clearing up of the skin. Or you may see breakouts on the skin as heavier toxins are being eliminated from there.

The middle passage may accelerate, finding more energy, fewer aches and pains, easier to resist previous temptations, fewer cravings for unhealthy foods, and new abilities, sensations, and vigor arise.

The end-game feels natural, awakening without having to inventory the damage, ready strength returned, a youthful awareness, appearance, and attitude, a determined focus as well as a sudden awareness when an endotoxin or exotoxin penetrates.

How long does each phase take place? It depends on your medical history, the nature of the illness to be addressed, and your own stick-to-it-ness with your healing protocol. It may be a week, or it may be a year. Is this a simple health issue or complex comorbidities compounded by years of neglect and an overload of metropolitan dust, diseases, and stress?

Look for small gains at first, and know that your body is healing, in its own time, and its own way. If it has taken 30 years or 40 years or 50 years to get to this point, it may take some time to heal.

The journey of a thousand miles begins with one step.

—Chinese Proverb

But you should know, Mother Nature is always righting herself....

Robin Hood Gets It Right Again.

Errol Flynn and Olivia De Havilland will always be the real Robin Hood and Lady Marion in the 1939 classic film, "The Adventures of Robin Hood." Even so, two of my favorite current Hollywood stars are Russell Crowe and Kate Blanchett. They starred in a recent, inventive version of the Robin Hood legends. While Robin still robs from the rich and gives to the poor, Lady Marion has gotten a real makeover in this retelling. She is the lady of the manor, holding together the Loxley earldom and estate, working side-by-side with hundreds of peasant farmers until her husband, Sir Loxley (too many details here; see the film) returns from the Crusades. We meet her in the farm fields, discussing the current, impoverished state common folk are experiencing while the king's tax collectors mirthfully punish people. Low on food, she nearly apologizes when telling a visitor she and the peasants are eating "....nettle soup and dandelion salad...." Staples of the Renaissance peasant, and if I had to choose two medicinal herbs to sustain me, they would be nettles and dandelion.

Nettles tea is like drinking a cup of vitamins. Dandelion roots clean out the liver and reset your clock. In Traditional Chinese Medicine, the first twelve hours of the day, the body is building up. In the second twelve hours of the day, the body is detoxifying. Both actions are supported by these two powerhouse herbs. In Renaissance Times, the peasants were the ones who regularly ate healthy foods: grass-fed beef, free roaming chicken, organic seasonal fruits, and freshly wildcrafted herbs from the fields. The kings and queens loaded up on honey-mead wine, denatured-white-flour, sailing vessels of sugar, pastries adorned with New World chocolate confections, and sauces smothered in "hot spices" from Asia. Those kings and queens were making worldly decisions with over-loaded-carbo-brain-fog, while the peasants danced merrily on nutrients found in the fields.

Tools for the Urban Herbalist—The Steps

Step 1: Owning Your Own Space

To be an urban herbalist, practicing in a cityscape of towering steel, fire escapes, overcrowded subways, the gamut from quaint shops to department stores, derailed tourists, wanderers sleeping in parks, taxis & Ubers drag racing the avenues, fast foods chasing international culinary fanfare, and uninvited in-laws along with uninformed friends, you have to own your own space.

When I was in my 20s, defining my life and knowing I would rather be convinced than defeated, I read an interesting quote: "The more powerful you are, the stronger your enemies will be." One American cultural trait we have around sharing a meal with family, friends, or even a business lunch, is the idea that when someone has a healthy plate of food, everyone eating SAD (Standard American Diet) gets to take shots *at the person who is eating healthy.*

"You don't have any fun, do you?"

"Is that all you're having?"

"Don't you want some bacon?"

"Pass her the French fries."

Many of us are up against a plethora of nagging health issues: Lyme's disease, ovarian cancer, IBS, debilitating asthma, ADD/ADHD, autism, chronic stress, obesity, neurodivergence, PTSD, brain fog, chronic lethargy, caffeine overload, allergies from A-Z, dismal pain, and recovery from alcohol and drug abuse. In the 21st century, we have advanced, Western medicine at our disposal, yet the issues are still here, and working on them means eating better foods.

When we dig deeper, a number of chronic, complex health issues began by a bombardment of medications and denatured foods. Many of us, currently and historically, have been helped by our herbal allies, and there are books, testimonials, scientific studies, and shared experiences to confirm this progress.

Then, somehow, family, friends, and community resist this unanticipated hope. So the first issue for self-healing is *to own your own space*.

When you know choosing healthy food practices is right because you are feeling good results in your own body, you are correct. You can say:

"I'm taking a self-care day."

"I'd rather not talk about that right now."

"You want me to _____ , and I'm not going to do that."

"Yes, I heard what you said the first time."

"I know what I experienced, and you can't convince me otherwise."

"I'm not responding to unhealthy choices which will undermine my recovery and good health."

"This is what I'm having."

"I have food allergies, and nothing else, thank you."

"I'm not having any ham (or whatever food dish someone suggests)."

The food you choose is part of your own space. You don't have to eat the same things, in the same quantities, or even at the same time, as other people.

Keep remembering how wonderful you'll feel when your body is detoxed, fortified, and humming along.

Step 1 1/2:
The Buying Committee

Holistic Moms, an eminent organization with a tender mission, helps educate moms (and dads) about "holistic parenting and green living." Members meet together to share information. I interviewed the founder of HolisticMoms.

Dime con quien andas,
y te dire quien eres.
(Tell me with whom you walk,
and I'll tell you who you are.)

—Spanish proverb

org, Dr. Nancy Peplinsky, on my radio show, The Urban Herbalist, and she told me an important story off-air during the commercial break which I later asked her to share on-air. When she first began meeting with the mothers she'd connected to in the waiting room of her pediatrician, they traded holistic tips on childcare. These mothers also shared how pressured they felt by *their own families* to stop using holistic practices with their children. Family members were urging them to give their kids more drugs and ditch the honey and chamomile tea. These holistic moms now found themselves giving each other support for practicing alternative health methods.

There are some unique American organizations that deserve a shout-out. *Alcoholics Anonymous* is the granddaddy of all the 12-step programs. AA initiated the brilliant idea of alcoholics meeting together with other alcoholics to listen, acknowledge, and support one another as each individual worked on his or her issues. Bill W. and Bob S. originally met in 1935 in Akron, Ohio to discuss their drinking habits and personal turmoil. And it worked. Having another fellow traveler *listen and hear* the traveler's own experiences has made all the difference to a person in recovery. The twelve-step format has been so successful, it has begat other 12-step programs including:

- ACA: Adult Children of Alcoholics

- Al-Anon/Alateen: for friends and families of alcoholics

- CA: Cocaine Anonymous

- CoDA: Co-Dependents Anonymous

- FA: Families Anonymous, for relatives and friends of addicts

- FAA: Food Addicts Anonymous

- GA: Gamblers Anonymous

- Gam-Anon/Gam-A-Teen: for friends and family members of problem gamblers

- NA: Narcotics Anonymous

- OA: Overeaters Anonymous

- SLAA: Sex and Love Addicts Anonymous

Notice there are groups for the families and friends of people in recovery. While it's not readily acceptable to some families with entrenched dynamics, the blueprint of family dynamics will have to change for the 12-stepper to recover.

Forming new habits affects the gameboard of family relationships (more perhaps that a new marriage or a new baby?). Those family dynamics must be part of the equation to reach your goal. With whom do you live? Or with whom do you speak every day? How well do you and your partner communicate? Do you have children you eat with every day? Children's eating habits tend to dominate family meals, so meal planning with young children is usually limited to a child's palate. Will objections be raised when you announce you will eat differently from your family? Will voices be raised? Will there be "a vote" about whether you are "allowed" to eat differently?

When someone returns home after a drug or alcohol rehab center, the center often advises as part of recovery that the person should stay away from his/her family of origin or even move out of the old neighborhood, so the person doesn't fall backwards. Some family members left behind would rather poke at the person in recovery instead of changing their own dysfunctional habits. (Twelve-step programs clearly define "enablers.") With alcohol and drugs, every 12-step program will tell you to stop using the substance. It's trickier around the issues of food and health because you can't stop eating. So your whole committee has to go along with you, or at least back off, or maybe be left behind.

When still a teenager, I visited my cousins in another state who took me to lunch at their friend's house. Their friend's sister and father joined us that day. The friend, Susie, wanted to lose 30 pounds, so she had put

> When you're serious about
> your dream:
>
> Be ready to be alone.
> Be ready to be laughed at.
> Be ready to be doubted.
> Be ready to be criticized.
> Be ready to be misunderstood.
> Be ready to lose many people.
>
> #millionairesteps

herself on a diet. While we were eating big, thick sweetened ham and smoked turkey sandwiches with chips, fries, and pickles on the table (this was before I learned about herbs and nutrition), Susie was eating some pre-cooked shrimp, no sauce, and a small salad of lettuce and carrots, with lemon juice dressing. She quietly placed her food on the table while we passed plates and piled on mayo. Sitting at the head of the table, Susie's father's remarked, "You think that's gonna work?" When people are reminded of their own self-absorbed/self-made limitations, they'll resort to almost anything to distract the conversation. He glared at Susie, who turned red, and waited. (Was he waiting for an apology?) I noticed the father could stand to lose about 40 pounds himself. Susie's sister was about Susie's size, yet Susie had had the courage to begin dieting. The father wouldn't stop. As my cousins tried to engage the girls in a discussion about going to the beach, the father just kept throwing out snide remarks. "She thinks if she eats shrimp, she's gonna be a model." "Who feels full after eating *that?*" "She's gonna gain it all back." I already felt the tug of what would become a major metaphysical theme in my life about directing my own path, so I saw this as an opportunity to serve others by example. I said to the father, "How long have you lived in this house?" Since I was a qualified stranger, I could ask these elongated "getting-to-know-you-questions" without looking out of place. The father immediately responded, "Twenty years." I replied, "Oh, so you planned ahead for your family to grow up here?" Pleased that *his efforts* were being noticed, he said yes, and I kept asking him how the neighborhood had changed over the years. I was a still a kid, didn't know how to name all of this, but I kept this guy occupied until everyone finished eating. He needed distraction from belittling Susie, since her self-discipline mirrored back to him his own insecurities. I caught Susie's eye and could see she was grateful. My two cousins looked relieved. Today, I would confront an adult like that for bullying his daughter in front of her friends and might even ask him to defend his own food choices. Or I'd hold court with stories of the resistance I experienced from others when I first started on my kitchen table in Greenwich Village, spread with leaves and flowers and roots. Ah, but that's a discussion for another day...

Get your whole buying committee on board before you start cooking with medicinal herbs and eating better, or get a new buying committee. You don't need mealtimes that look like Susie's.

> Happiness is made of small things.
>
> Identify limiting beliefs and then identify your goals.
>
> Stick to your goals...

Step 2: Your Turn: Write Down Your Medical History

Before a consultation, I ask each client to write down his/her medical history. Most people can easily remember big things—"pneumonia in early 20s and broke my right leg skiing in Colorado, age 32." Yet there are more items to add to your personal inventory.

Homework: *Kindly write every drug you have ever taken in your life, every surgery/medical procedure you've had done, and any other illnesses you have experienced, especially within the last ten years.*

Sample Drug List:

- as a child from 6-10, a lot of penicillin every time I got the flu.
- meds as a teen for acne (don't remember the names).
- birth control, Lisina, from March 2001-December 2019.
- different diuretics before menstrual cycle.
- Flonase/respiratory gets worse, since age of 25.
- heavy aspirin for migraines since the age of 26, 3-4 migraines a month.
- sometimes Advil or Excedrin for migraines.
- antibiotics for Lyme's disease, 2008 and again in 2020.
- antibiotics for Covid 2021.
- Lipitor, 2004-present.
- six vaccinations before photography safari abroad
- Zoloft from June 2014 to September 2021.

Most people have 10-30 items on their lists.

(Sample) History List:

- tonsils out at age 9.
- broken foot, age 14.
- bad acne from ages 15-22.
- chills, horrible cramps for each period, age 13 on.
- fungal skin infection after vacation to Southeast Asia, age 28.
- little headaches beginning at 14 to migraines beginning in 20s, getting worse.
- football tackled in college; concussion.
- appendectomy, age 33.
- severe allergies after my first child was born, age 35.
- second child, age 39.
- colonoscopy, age 45.
- severe runny nose and sore throat when I started working in new office building, 2 years ago.

- 4 stents implanted, age 57

Most people have 6-15 items on their lists.

You can take a piece of paper, write down everything you remember currently, and then put the paper on a "daily altar." A daily altar is a spot like your most-often-used kitchen counter or on top of your favorite dresser. As you walk by it for a couple of days, you'll begin remembering this-and-that for each list. (Most people need additional time for remembering so many details.) These lists are valuable tools. When analyzing yourself, begin to see patterns or clues about how and when your body became vulnerable or started to falter.

Health tip: As part of your own inventory, it's important to understand *your* innate immune system. When did you *not* get sick, when others in your family were falling ill? Where has your body always exceled? Which food groups does your body respond to the quickest? Which remedies have you tried (especially when younger) that hardly affected you? It's a good time to ask granny what she remembers health wise about you as a child, moreover, about everyone else on the family tree.

Step 3: Live Inside Your Body/How Do You Feel?

When you wake up, ask yourself, "How do I feel?" Unless the average person has a terrible flu, is pregnant, recovering from surgery, or has a rare tropical disease picked up traipsing around a flowering Pacific island, most people just get up and go. But then, many people stumble through their days drinking coffee, expresso, umpteen-hour energy shots, and later in the afternoon, take L-theanine, a glass of wine, or a little CBD (full cannabis spectrum?) to mellow out. This does not gauge the foods this person has eaten for the day—enough nutrients? no nutrients? excipients? fillers?

genetically modified foods (GMOs)? special diet? Many people don't recognize the signals the body sends out constantly. I knew a relatively young mother (44) who was diagnosed with breast cancer the day before Thanksgiving, and by December 23, she died. (Her daily intake was a pack of cigarettes and a bag of supermarket cookies. What signals from her body did she overlook?)

Take a baseline of your body daily:
- Does my head ache?
- Do I need a bowel movement?
- Can I easily stretch and bend?
- Am I craving any particular food? coffee? sugar? salt? more meat? more vegetables?
- Can I breathe easily?

Step 4: Do These in Whatever Order Feels Right:
- Commit time to studying. See the List of Works Cited for this book; read several of those. You can begin with just two pages a day.

- Spend some money on dried bulk herbs, a pot to boil water in, and a tea strainer.

- If you want to, grow some of your own herbs. Starting with a flower pot on your fire escape is smart for an urban herbalist. A friend just showed me a flower pot that comes with its own grow-light. Perfect for the apartment/city dweller, a favorite plant can be nurtured individually inside. Just remember, it takes a growing season to sprout and bloom, so if you need an herb *today,* buy it from the store. Also, you may want to use herbs that cannot be grown in your climate, or you just may not have enough space to grow everything you want to try. Buying bulk herbs, instead of growing them or foraging them, is okay.

Mother Nature knows you may not have the forest resources of our ancestors; the idea is simply to get started.

- Allergy testing: One very important medical service is **food allergy testing**. Even if you were tested ten years ago, do it again. Bodies change for all kinds of reasons: moving more than seven degrees longitude or seven degrees latitude, having a baby, a radical change in diet (i.e., becoming vegan or returning to meat-eating), body traumas, surgeries, stress, or coping with a severe, long-term illness. These changes affect your body systems, so get tested. Everybody is allergic to molds and dust; tell the doctor you want to be tested for *food allergies*. After getting the test results, cut out *everything* you're allergic to. Yes, easier said than done. However, once you eliminate allergens, your body responds wonderfully! Elimination of allergens usually results in increased energy, greater concentration, sustained stamina, and a better sense of well-being. Your body chi won't be exhausted protecting itself against invading pathogens any more.

Thought for the day: Cave people just ate their herbs. Today, people who want to practice antiquarian herbalism are told "to just go out and gather them," but not everyone can do that. I heard one gardener on a webinar tell everyone to simply open up his/her backdoor and "go get them, even go to the park." (Not a great idea for city life if everyone is tearing out plants from the precious, limited, preserved park space.) There is this popular "holistic" idea out there that everyone dedicate time all week to foraging and making tinctures to be apportioned like a druggist in a lab coat. This gardener also instructed everyone to use herbs in a phytoherbalism way, to make tinctures, salves, and electuaries, quantifying the dosages. It is ironic that the expectation is that everyone can simply live off the land, but "live with a dispensary." The urban herbalist gathers herbs from stores, online, and from window boxes, but uses herbs like cave people. Medical vegetables can be nibbled, sauteed, roasted, baked, tossed, chopped, simmered, sipped, stewed, and brewed. They are the plants for our daily diets.

Why do vegetables not taste better?

Before our envelope taste buds were pushed, with white sugar in tomato sauces, brown sugar toppings on baked salmon, candied pecans for salads, and honey-coated breakfast cereals to gyrate our early mornings, we had a taste for the green leafy things in the forest. Roots and bark were fine, and stems and flowers retained their own sweetness. It was only when the trade routes opened up from across Asia and the New World that the royal court master chefs began experimenting with novel ingredients, most noticeably sugar. The regal request became "make it sweeter." No court-appointed doctor had any scientific evidence about palate derangement, heart disease, and IBS development on hand. What was fit for the king must be fit for the surfs, and so the new cooking trends tended towards sweet pies and stimulating sauces. Sugar as a food stuff was industrialized in the 1800s, and crowded city life looked for relief anywhere, most notably through drinking and desserts. As Western culture became indulgently accustomed to the candied dulcitude being served, taste buds started rejecting the mineral content in dark, green leafy vegetables. A favorite Instagram post I saw was of a two-year-old little girl, barefoot, holding her young, pet chicken under her left arm, and wandering peacefully around the raised vegetable garden beds her parents put up. She casually plucked off kale leaves to nibble on. How nice it was that there were no adults squawking, "How can she do that? Oh, do you really like those?" No one was limiting her instincts. She was showing us what a natural childhood really looks like.

Current Statistics

"Incidence rates for deaths directly attributable to medical care gone awry haven't been recognized in any standardized method for collecting national statistics," says Martin Makary, M.D., M.P.H., professor of surgery at the Johns Hopkins University School of Medicine and an authority on health reform. "The medical coding system was designed to maximize billing for physician services, not to collect national health statistics, as it is currently being used." https://www.hopkinsmedicine.org/

- Fast Facts: 10 percent of all U.S. deaths are now due to medical error.

- The third-highest cause of death in the U.S. is medical error.

- Medical errors are an under-recognized cause of death. (www.hopkinsmedicine.org).

- "Then, using **hospital** admission rates from 2013, they extrapolated that based on a total of 35,416,020 **hospitalizations,** 251,454 deaths stemmed from a medical error, which the researchers say now translates to 9.5 percent of all deaths each year

No "silver bullet" for modern life.

There is no "silver bullet" for complex health issues, which many Americans face today. The combination of environmental pollutants, an overload of synthetic drugs, debilitating stress, toxic relationships—at home and on the job, denatured foods, and the overpopulation of the earth, have led to the expressions of illnesses previously undefined by Mother Nature 200,000 years ago when she sat in the Garden of Eden, sipping tea and designing our bodies for living on this planet. The plants have already adapted; it is our turn to adapt now.

in the United States. (https://www.hopkinsmedicine.org/news/media/releases)

> "You never step into the same stream twice."
>
> —Heraclitus

- "They also found that more diagnostic error claims were rooted in **outpatient** care than inpatient care, **(68.8 percent vs. 31.2 percent)** but inpatient diagnostic errors were more likely to be lethal (48.4 percent vs. 36.9 percent)." (https://www.hopkinsmedicine.org/news/media/releases)

- "While the new study looked only at a subset of claims—those that rose to the level of a malpractice payout—researchers estimate the number of patients suffering misdiagnosis-related, potentially preventable, significant permanent injury or death annually in the United States ranges from 80,000 to 160,000." (https://www.hopkinsmedicine.org/news/media/releases)

- When asked how many people died from an herb, neither the https://www.hopkinsmedicine.org/news/media/releases nor the https://www.cdc.gov/nchs/fastats/deaths.htm had any statistics.

- An herbal plant is not a manufactured remedy, with additives, excipients, and small quantities of secret drugs that may have been added by overseas companies who don't operate by the guidelines of the American FDA. While every person must exercise caution, the facts are showing herbal teas have a proven record of less adverse events occurring.

Omnium-Gatherum of Sage Advice

- In Traditional Chinese Medicine, the client doesn't pay until the client feels better.

- In an appointment with a doctor, the patient has only a short time for that consultation. The requirements of allopathic medicine and insurance companies are that doctors see many patients in a day, turning each patient into a series of billing codes. There are many good doctors who are frustrated by this arrangement as well. When someone makes an appointment with an herbalist, the person usually confers with that holistic practitioner for over an hour and gets to tell his/her whole story. *The whole story helps to get the whole answer.*

- Plant medicine subscribes to the innate wisdom of nature; let the healing process work.

- Even as a child, I loved seeing plants, all plants, springing up through the cracks in sidewalks. It was the earth spirit saying hello.

- Get a group together and go to a health food store. Examine brands, read labels, ask the salespeople questions. Talk to other people in the aisles, especially the ones who've put a few bottles of nutraceuticals and a few boxes of tea bags into their carts. They already have a good idea about what to do.

- Get a group together and practice cooking your recipes with medicinal herbs. Blend teas and share stories. This formula worked, that formula didn't. Ask questions about kitchen tools, cutting shears, and measurements. Ask about the service at one health food store or from an online, bulk herb supplier. Ask how much sunlight that plant received and in which direction his/her fire escape was facing when the plant was growing. North? South?

- In a circle with other practitioners, sit together, season after season, and discuss the pains, symptoms, setbacks, strides, and victories you've seen in yourself and others, again and again and again; that is your commencement.

- Walk through a garden with a child. Follow a child's wonder. See plants blossoming and butterflies flutter by. Remember that connection.

- Walk down a city block. Find a dandelion poking up in the large institutional pots placed unceremoniously in front of imposing skyscraper entrances. Look for plants sprouting up between side-walk cracks, in the cobblestoned beds around trees, and fighting for light in city lots, highway meridians, and on the shoulder of the road. Smile at them. Remember their names. Honor their courage and earth spirit.

- Go to an old people's home. They give value to the wrinkles they've earned. It's a bit humbling, learning about old remedies, and you get more than you give.

- Weekend, internet classes hand out certificates on herbology, without apprenticeship nor riding the high and lows of a dominating disease. The certifications are usually about foraging on 40 acres of land, and then practicing phytoherbalism, an imitation of Western allopathic medicine, with tinctures and extracts. The mothercraft of urban herbalism is to gather herbs available from apothecaries and flower pots, and then practice ethnobotany, the employment of the herbs as food in the manner of how their actions correspond to body systems. It is acting in rhythm with nature.

- Try each herb on yourself, then blend teas for family and friends.

- Nobody knows everything. In college, a favorite sociology professor said, "Most important skill coming up—*knowing how to learn.*"

- Be in nature with an animal, off-leash, uncaged. Notice the way they drink in the grass, trees, flowers, and climbing every rock is an adventure. That spirit of exploration used to be ours, too.

- Cook the same meal on a gas range, over an electric stove, on a grill, and on top of a camp fire with wood you had to gather. Observe the ingredients, texture of the foods, how the flavors change, and how much appreciation you have for the dish each time it is prepared. Understand how much of yourself is in there.

- Grazing is an acceptable way of eating. Sitting together in groups several times daily as the "proper" way to eat is, again, founded on distant, cultural habits. Some diets call for six short meals a day, which is actually closer to the grazing habits of our cave ancestors. Planning to share a major meal daily with loved ones is fine, *and* give yourself permission to nibble when you want to.

- Someone remarked how inappropriate it is seeing a mother with a week-old baby wheeling it around a noisy, unpredictable mall. This attests to the fact that in the 21st century, "progress" for most city dwellers equals being out-of-touch with the subtle energies influencing our bodies. All living beings have auras or energy fields that are electro-magnetic, talismanic, and when best encountered, enchanting. This energy is always vibrating and being exchanged with other people, animals, plants, and places. The energy your child is exposed to will certainly influence that child and even your pets. (Why do so many people spend their dog-walking time on their cell phones?) While conglomerates and aerodynamic physicists have yet to figure out quantifying this energy exchange, healing shamen have long recognized this flow and supported the value of imbuing one's self with the auras and sensuous spirits of nature. (Ever notice how renewed a city dweller feels when returning from a vacation at the beach or in the mountains?) The more we work with plants, the complete, whole roots, leaves, twigs, bark, berries, seeds, and flowers, the more we take on the characteristics of being natural, centered, and live harmoniously with nature and other people.

- All herbal teas, without any sugars or milk (dairy or otherwise) make excellent fertilizers for your plants. Even if you are watering the flower pots on your fire escape (a favorite summer hang-out place for urban herbalists), your plants will welcome the nutrients and green energy from their herbal allies.

- When I began looking into alternative health in the 1970s, there was no health food industry. No Whole Foods, no granola bars, no naturopaths, no indie book stores, no Amazon, and no meet-ups for kindred spirits to find their tribe. I've watched the health food industry grow up and spread out. Talk about grass roots. By word of mouth and without commercials. That's saying something.

The Lovely Couple from China

When unpacking delivery crates in my health food store one morning, an entire Greyhound tourist bus en route to West Point stopped on my street. It was in Highland Falls, the town where West Point is located, and visitors from around world came to experience this piece of history. Sometimes I felt more like a hostess than a shopkeeper. A lovely couple from China came in that day, and in careful, broken, English managed to convey that the wife was carsick from the long bus ride they'd taken from New York City to get to the Hudson Valley. Somehow, they made the bus driver understand they didn't want a drugstore; they wanted an apothecary. I smiled as I took down one of my gallon, brown-glass apothecary jars and got out a piece of crystalized ginger. They looked curious. They asked me something with a Chinese word, "Is (Chinese word)?" My turn to look puzzled. The wife bit into the ginger and began to smile. She knew what it was and was on her way to feeling better. They began pointing to other apothecary jars and telling me the names of the herbs in Chinese. Somehow, through laughter and multiloquence, we traded remedy use, asked questions, and connected like only travelers do. We were sharing how to heal. The husband took pictures of his wife and I posing in my bay window, loaded with holistic health books and plants. Smiling and bowing, they waved when they left. A good day in the shop.

In Renaissance times, labor was cheap, and herbs were expensive. Plants had to be carried across mountains and deserts and hostile territories, preserved with scant water and a brief, daily dose of sunlight. Today, herbs are cheap, with culinary cuttings in every garden store and supermarket, and labor is oh, so expensive.

Edinburgh is an esteemed, medieval European city dating back to 1130. Quaint, grand, intimate, and imposing, these city dwellers have long honored the intellectualism of the European court, the maneuvers of Machiavelli, and the favorable benison of the Scottish countrymen. Unyoked because of their distance from London, they've a heritage that allows them to cherry-pick what they choose to learn. The Scots care about their history and anyone who has contributed to it. Sashaying around Edinburgh one afternoon, we came upon an antiquarian book store, and I couldn't get inside fast enough. Lots of dusty novels and crinkled mariners' maps. One stuffed cardboard box had to be dragged out from under the mantelpiece. There were individual pages from 1600s books, discarded by printers for flaws in the hand stitching. Huzzah, I found two original materia medica pages from Gerard's 1633 edition. They're hanging above my desk right now as I type. Motherwort, Basil (*Bafill*), Stinging Nettle (flinging Nettle), and Pennyroyal (Pennie Royall) are the materia medica entries, and they're uncannily accurate for today. There were three materia medica written during the Renaissance that are still referenced today: John Gerard's *The Herball of Generall Historie of Plantes* (1597), Nicolas Culpepper's *Complete Herbal & English Physician* (1652), and John Parkinson's "*Theatrum Botanicum* (1640). What incredible knowledge was already gathered and written down for us.

I was lucky enough to spend nearly four years doing primary research with Parkinson's *Theatrum Botanicum* (1640). His many painstakingly assembled, extended descriptions of the herbs were more than a labor of love by the queen's herbarist (not herbalist; *herbarist, old English*). Each plant's appearance, virtues, and harvesting requirements were noted in great detail. In times of need, the gatherer had to devise a healing protocol with whatever was on hand, relying on her memory of this vast compendium. These were survival skills, nurtured by the frugal goodwives who skillfully improvised in the moment.

Embrace that self-healing goes beyond food, water, and exercise.

Meditation, prayer, walking, being in nature, reading metaphysical and spiritual literature, volunteering, cleaning out closets, exploring art, watching favorite old movies, and living with wholesome, healthy people all contribute to self-healing. Additionally, you can include acupuncture treatments, chiropractic adjustments, sound healing, somatic therapy, meditation, reiki, hiking in nature, and workouts. All these things work in tandem.

The New Wave of Ingredients

- Kombucha—called a "health elixir." Kombucha tea is a fermented drink made with tea, sugar, bacteria, and yeast.

- Kimchi—a traditional Korean side dish of salted and fermented vegetables, such as napa cabbage and Korean radish.

- Gomasio—sesame salt.

- Umeboshi plums (or umeboshi paste)—plumes pickled in brine.

- Kuzu—a starch from the root of the kudzu plant with an alkalizing effect.

These are found in a health food store.

Dieting

Usually "dieting" means eating a regimen of food different from one's previous routine in order to lose weight. When the regimen is over, even if the weight has been lost, many people return to their old eating habits, and the weight comes back. When simple steps are taken to shift some eating habits *and social habits*, gently, into healthier habits, as well as blend medicinal herbs into one's daily meals, the body will find its own, healthy, slimmed down weight.

While some advocate for "no soy milk," it's usually based on the average American shopper having so many soy-substitute fillers that interfere with the endocrine system. When not loaded up on fast food burgers, oil-soaked fries, and big bomb soda explosions, the body more easily absorbs, stores, apportions, and utilizes the myriad of nutrients taken in daily. Occasional soy milk, soybeans, or soy burgers can be enjoyed anytime.

M.'s Mothercraft Crop-Rotation Theory of Healing

One thing is for sure: crop rotation really works. Utilized as early as 6,000 BC, Middle Eastern farmers rotated their crops to improve soil, reduce pests, eliminate weeds, and increase biodiversity. Crop rotation was later practiced by farmers in ancient Rome, Greece, and China. A natural habitat needs variety to remain fresh, and our own bodies respond to a crop rotation of foods, remedies, exercise, and mental challenge. Likewise, when wandering and reading the forested landscape, gatherers encountered new plants, which in turn provided additional nutrients. Our bodies were designed to store, sort out, recycle, uptake, and eliminate the assemblage of foodstuffs the ancients ingested.

Illness in the body is not stagnant. It shifts, reacts, explodes, transforms, and subsides. There is an arc of the illness of which the practitioner must be aware and respond to; there should be daily, weekly, or monthly adjustments necessary to someone's healing protocol. Think of having a cold. The first day may be a scratchy throat. The second day may be chills and a sniffle. By the third day, it's sneezing, coughing, and a loss of appetite. The fourth day could intensify everything from day three and include a headache, insomnia, and a mild fever. Then the cold might break, and on the fifth day, the fever goes down, the headache is gone, and sleep is no problem. For the next two to three days, other symptoms taper off. (In Traditional Chinese Medicine, the apothecary-doctor tells the patient to come back the next day to see which herbs the person needs after the results of the previous day's herbs.) Likewise, with competing co-morbidities, each participating illness must be monitored, with adjustments to treatments when appropriate. For example, if the immune system is being supported, you might begin working with golden seal for a two weeks, then go to pau d'arco for a month, and lastly work with coltsfoot and damiana. (Other herbs and supplements can address other body systems during this time.) It helps the body to shift and "taste" a different strategy.

Beginning Protocols: Let's say a woman is working on her **chronic period cramps concurrently with springtime allergies**. The springtime allergies take precedence, because they are seasonal and immediate; therefore, she can begin with three or four days of respiratory herbs and intestinal healing. As her menstrual cycle approaches, she can begin herbs to help regulate and ease menstrual discharge. The menstrual herbs can begin a week ahead of the first day of her period, as well as the respiratory herbs, as needed. When various treatments are rotated, a tolerance to the essential antidotes should not happen. The longer you work with herbs, the more immersed you are, the more attuned to nature, and the better you know your body, the easier mothercrafting your crop-rotation will become.

Inflammation, antioxidant, and joint support: no nightshades:

- Breakfast—scrambled eggs, with spinach, turmeric, celery salt, pepper, and two capsules of turmeric.
- Snack—10:00 a.m., coconut yogurt with devil's claw, dandelion, ginger, blueberries.
- Lunch— a salad, including artichoke, cleavers, dandelion.
- Dinner—prepared chicken dish, white willow bark. Two or three cups of your choice of tea daily.

Mental alertness, memory function:

- Breakfast—smoothie with blueberries, strawberries, fenugreek, burdock, ginseng or ginkgo.
- Snack—gluten-free crackers, almond butter mixed with bacopa and bee pollen.
- Lunch—burrito with ginseng or gingko.
- Dinner—prepared fish with lemon balm, yarrow, and two capsules of dandelion. Two or three cups of your choice of tea daily.

Immune support and liver function:

- Breakfast—smoothie with papaya, bananas, spinach, nettles, pau d'arco.
- Snack—coconut yogurt with spirulina, coconut shreds.
- Lunch—sandwich wrap with milk thistle, burdock.
- Dinner—prepared chicken dish with milk thistle, pau d'acro. Two or three cups of your choice of tea daily, the last cup = oat straw or lemon balm.

Should using a variety of herbs throughout the day feel like a lot to organize, then just begin adding two herbs daily to your foods. As you become acclimated to supplementing your meals, blending in this variety becomes easier and easier.

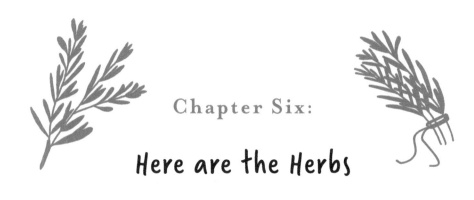

Chapter Six:

Here are the Herbs

Glossary of the Actions and Effects of the Materia Medica

- Abortifacient—Causes a miscarriage or spontaneous abortion.

- Adaptogen—Well known in China and the East, the doctrine of preventative medicine: an action that improves the body's adaptability to a health issue.

- Alterative—Positively alters/converts a morbid disease to a healthier state.

- Analgesic—A pain reliever, without causing unconsciousness.

- Anaphrodisiac—Decreases excessive sexual desires.

- Anesthetic—Impels unconsciousness or acts as an anesthesia. (Taber's)

- Anodyne—Quiets hypersensitivity of nerves. (Taber's)

- Antacid—Can neutralize acidity in stomach and intestines.

- Anthelmintic—Useful in treating parasitic intestinal worms.

- Antianemic—Increases red blood cells or hemoglobin in the blood.

Regulating 101: Scientific inquiry into the efficacy of herbs

Every plant is made up of chemicals. Herbs are plants with large quantities of chemicals that especially contribute nutritional as well as culinary benefits for humans. They work for people as medicines, foods, flavorings, and dyes. Scientists are always pulling matter apart, and, in their quest for finding cures, have bisected, divided, isolated, analyzed, and evaluated all the chemicals in medicinal vegetables. The Himalaya Drug Company, begun in 1930 as an Ayurvedic herb company in India, has clinically tested, as per chemical drug standards, much of the Ayurvedic materia medica. Their scientific studies are used globally by scientists, doctors, and nutraceutical brand makers. Likewise, the German E-Commission Monographs were first originated in 1978 by the advisory board of the Federal Institute for Drugs and Medical Devices. The German E-Commission provides scientific data for the approval of substances, plants, and products previously used in traditional, folk, and herbal medicine. The commission became known outside of Germany in the 1990s for compiling and publishing 380 monographs evaluating the safety, efficacy, and medicinal qualities of herbs for licensed medical prescribing in Germany. Their work was made public in the United States when the American Botanical Council translated the monographs into English. Additionally, numerous scientific studies are done round the world to quantify the medicinal constituents of herbs as well as definitive dosages for prescribing purposes. A wide range of industry periodicals publish these studies which provide the basis for expansion of nutraceutical product lines within the health food industry. One significant, annual convention is the Integrative Healthcare Symposium held in New York City. Open only to doctors, scientists, and licensed health practitioners, this symposium globally draws in top medical researchers reporting the latest, extended, scientific studies. Participants delve into the published analyses involving the interactions between herbs and medications. I have always welcomed attending this particular event. It's so joyful talking to medical doctors who want to embrace a natural approach for antiseptics and antidotes. Historic folk medicine has been validated and reached the 21st century.

- Antiarthritic—Relieves symptoms of arthritis and gout.

- Antiasthmatic—Relieves symptoms of asthma.

- Antibacterial—Hinders the growth and reproduction of bacteria.

- Anticatarrhal—Quells inflammation of mucus membranes, preventing development of mucus.

- Antidepressive—Can alleviate depression and encourage a positive mood.

- Antidiabetic —Treats diabetes.

- Antiemetic—Reduces nausea and prevents against vomiting.

- Antifungal—Subdues fungal infections of the scalp, skin, and nails.

- Anti-inflammatory—Decreases inflammatory response.

- Antilithic—Helps prevent gravel or stones in the urinary system.

- Antimicrobial—Kills microorganisms, bacteria, fungi, algae, and viruses as well as quells further growth.

- Antineoplastic—Addresses treatment of cancer.

- Antioxidant—Reduces free radical damage.

- Antiperiodic—Prevents regular reoccurrence for illness with high fever, i.e. malaria.

- Antipyretic—Causes the hypothalamus to override a prostaglandin-induced increase in temperature, reduces fever.

- Antirheumatic—Therapeutic for inflammatory arthritis.

- Antiseptic—Acts to prevent decay, putrefaction, or sepsis.

- Antispasmodic—Relieves or prevents "fits" and "spasms."

- Antiviral—Inhibits or kills a virus or its ability to replicate.

- Aperient—A mild medicine or food that acts as a laxative.

- Aphrodisiac—Stimulates sexual desire.

- Aromatic—The agreeable aroma (from volatile essential oils) can induce good moods, stimulate digestion, open clogged nasal passages, or expectorate the lungs.

- Astringent—An agent acting to bind or constrict body tissues, usually a topical application; checks hemorrhages, secretions, or may cause mouth to feel dry.

- Bitters—Stimulate the digestive tract including saliva, gastric juices, bile, pancreatic juices, and intestinal juices.

- Cardiac depressant —Decreases the heart's action.

- Cardiac stimulant —Increases the heart's action.

- Carminative—Rich in volatile oils, known to soothe the gut walls, helps remove gas, and encourages peristalsis.

- Cholagogue—Stimulates bile flow.

- Circulatory stimulant—Increases circulation.

- Demulcent—Soothes and protects irritated mucous membranes.

- Deodorant—Diminishes foul odors.

- Diaphoretic—Promotes sweating, which can clear the skin, reduce fevers, eliminate toxins, and quiet aching joints.

- Disinfectant—Kills bacteria and germs.

- Diuretic—Increases the flow of urine.

- Emetic—Promotes vomiting.

- Emmenagogue—Can assist menstrual flow.

- Emollient—Will soften and soothe the skin, restore moisture, acts to repair damaged skin; much the same as internally used demulcents.

- Errhines —Causes increased nasal secretions.

- Exhilarant—Stimulates mental activity and acts to uplift spirits and elevate mood.

- Expectorant—Removes excess mucus from lungs and throat, treating respiratory issues.

- Febrifuge—Lessens a fever.

- Fomentation—The application of hot, moist substances on the body to ease pain; the material applied: poultice.

- Galactagogue—Increases milk flow in a lactating woman.

- Hepatic—Helps to strengthen, detoxify, and aid the work of the liver; increases bile flow.

- Hypnotic—Causes insensibility to pain or can induce sleep.

- Hypoglycemic—Acts to lower blood sugar (also a condition in someone with low blood sugar).

- Hypotensive—Acts to decrease blood pressure; an anti-hypertensive.

- Immunomodulator—Raises immune system activity if there's a deficiency, or subdues excessive activity, as in an autoimmune disease.

- Laxative—Can induce bowel movements, loosen dried fecal matter.

- Litholitic—Acts to break down urinary stones.

- Lymphatic—Elevates the operation of lymph glands.

- Mucilant—A gelatinous plant substance that contains protein and polysaccharides and moistens.

- Mydriatic—Causes pupil dilation.

- Narcotic—Agent that depresses the central nervous system, thus relieving pain and producing sleep; but which in excessive doses, produces unconsciousness, stupor, coma, and possibly death...Most are habit forming. (Taber's)

- Nephritic—Benefits kidney problems.

- Nervine—Benefits and calms the nerves.

- Nutrients—Assimilated vitamins and minerals; de facto, for nourishing and healing our bodies. Classified herbs have, through empirical and scientific knowledge, numerous nutrients proven to deliver the healthy components of nutrition to our bodies for growth and repair.

- Oxytocic—Stimulates the contraction of uterine muscles or hastens childbirth.

- Pectoral—Benefits the respiratory system.

- Poultice—The application of hot, moist substances to the body to ease pain; the material applied in fomentation.

- Purgative—Stimulates the evacuation of the bowels, for cleansing, eliminating toxins, and alleviating migraines.

- Refrigerant—Induces the body to feel cool.

- Rubefacient—Hardly used now, yet at one time, a topical application that caused a dilation of the capillaries to increase blood circulation.

- Sedative—Subdues physical behavior and promotes a calming of the mind.

- Sialagogue—Induces the salivary glands activity.

- Stimulant—Elevates energy levels, by way of temporarily increasing circulation, alertness, endurance, productivity, mental activity, heart rate, and blood pressure. (Sustained use may overload the liver and brain.)

- Stomachic—Addresses stomach activity.

- Tonic—Nutrient-rich, these herbs strengthen body systems as well as decrease toxicity in our organs.

- Vasodilator—Relaxes cells within the vessel walls, particularly in the large veins. Vasoconstriction is the narrowing of blood vessels.

- Vermicides—Can expel intestinal worms.

- Vulnerary—Speeds up healing wounds, cuts, rashes, and skin eruptions.

Any herb that contains "officinalis" or "officinale" in its Latin name has an enduring history as a therapeutic medicine. These Latin-named medicinal plants were kept in stock by Renaissance apothecaries as drugs. They were recognized by the medical pharmacopoeia and delivered to the kings and queens.

The word "drug" comes from the Dutch word "droog" which means "dry" or "to dry." It references how ancient healers, apothecaries, and physicians would dry their plants before using them as medicines.

A "simple" was the term Renaissance apothecaries employed for *a single herb being used by itself.* "Simpling" was *the practice of using just one herb at a time.* Simpling is still valuable, because you learn how a particular herb affects your body. Learning includes designing your own simpling protocols as well as blending your own unique formulas.

A Wild Thyme in the City Materia Medica

Today herbs are usually put into one of two categories: culinary or medicinal. Historically, all herbs were *culinary* and eaten regularly by the tribe when gatherers brought them back from the day's foraging. Each person ate piecemeal from numerous plant sources, what we'd call today "multi-vitamin-mineral-super-foods." Because everyone regularly ate naturally, supporting all of his/her body systems (digestive, immune, cardio, respiratory, reproductive, etc.), people maintained a good balance of homeostasis. Today we call this "preventative" health.

The mothercrafting idea today is to continuously eat valuable, nutritious, medical vegetables every day, all day. The following definitions are primarily based on the work of Rosemary Gladstar, David Hoffman, David Winston, Peeka Trenkle, Arcus Flynn, Louise Tenney, Native American elders, antiquarian materia medica, historic, empirical research, and curated, current industry research. (See the List of Works Cited.)

The advice of an herbalist is never meant to supplant the diagnosis of a licensed medical doctor. Herbal information is meant to augment a sound, clinical protocol developed for the patient's highest and best needs.

Alfalfa (Medicagto sativa) leaves and flowers, native to Europe and introduced to North America by the Spaniards. Virtues: alterative, blood purifier, lymphatic. Alfalfa sprouts are a staple at most health food stores and farmers' markets. Containing equivalents of human estrogen, alfalfa assists with female conditions and assimilating proteins and nutrients. It's a systems' cleanser, infection fighter, breaks down poisonous carbon dioxide, and a rich food source of trace minerals. Can be used to aid recuperation from alcoholism and drug addictions.

Angelica (Angelica atropurpurea) roots and seeds, native to Europe. Virtues: sometimes employed as a remedy for the plague in Europe, Angelica addressed blood impurities, gas, heartburn, and digestion.

(Angelica archangelica) roots and leaves, native to the high mountains of Switzerland. Virtues: carminative, and useful for coughs, bronchitis, colds, influenza, and as a digestive aid.

Artichoke (Cynara cardunculus) flower, native to southern Europe. Virtues: anti-inflammatory, aperient, cholagogue, digestant, diuretic, hepatic. A common vegetable today, artichoke activates the gallbladder which aids in digestion. This therapeutic deals with digestive tract issues, dyspepsia, bloating, flatulence, and poor appetite. It supports regeneration of the liver and detoxification. Delightfully, it's still one food eaten in our culture with your fingers. Peeling off the "flower petals" of this edible thistle, from the bracts to the artichoke heart, and dipping them into a sauce is convivial, conversational, and a great way to introduce a child to healthy eating.

Astragalus (Astragalus membranaceus) root, native to China. Virtues: antiviral, antibacterial, anti-inflammatory, adaptogen, and immunostimulant. Activates the immune system and stimulates the body systems, especially the respiratory system. "Studies by the American Cancer Society show the positive effects of astragalus on the immune systems of cancer patients tested. Those patients undergoing radiation and chemotherapy recovered faster and lived longer if they took astragalus during treatment." (Tenney) Useful for the common cold, it has secondary applications to immune deficiencies, kidney, stress, and arthritis.

Bacopa (Bacopa monnieri) leaves and stems, native to Eastern India, Asia, and Australia. Virtues: antioxidant (to the brain), grounding, nervine, stimulant, enhances mental focus. Also known as Brahmi, Herb of Grace, it has a long-standing history in Ayurvedic herbalism for supporting mood, attention span, and focus. And it can assist learning while calming a restless mind; these twin actions are associated with resting a preoccupied mind and quieting the sensitive, excitability of an adolescent. In our overloaded, information age, it's not logical to think that anyone can keep up with the bombardment of social media and far outreaches of cyberspace. It seems this gentle little tropical wildflower has really come of age. One mother gave bacopa to her previously "spaced out" teenager, and he was able to center himself enough to complete his research paper.

Barberry (Berberis vularis) bark of the root and berries, native to Europe. Virtues: "Studies have found that berberine contains properties effective against a wide variety of bacteria, viruses and fungi and that berberine was more effective in treating some bacteria than a strong antibiotic." (Tenney) Antiseptic, anti-inflammatory, anti-microbial, promotes removal of morbid matter from the stomach and bowels, associated with nearly every gastrointestinal ailment, lymphatics, urinary tract and respiratory infection, a bitter tonic and antipyretic. "Increases intestinal secretions, hence finds a place in the treatment of atonic dyspepsia, torpid conditions of liver..." (Park, Davis, & Co.) Berberine, the primary alkaloid, is a potent antibiotic.

Bay (Laurus nobilis) leaves, native to the Mediterranean. Virtues: carminative, aromatic, stomachic. "Stimulant, narcotic, astringent." (Parke, Davis & Co.) Encourages digestion, tones and strengthen the digestive system, and expels wind. (Every recipe feels exotic when bay is added!)

Bee pollen, native to bees, found everywhere. Virtues: around 40 percent protein, with amino acids, enzymes, essential fatty acids, vitamins, and minerals, all gathered by local bees from their local pollen to make their local honey. Ancient Greeks recognized that marathon runners increased speed and endurance when consuming bee pollen. Each considered a complete food, bee pollen and honey are highly regarded for assisting newcomers with acclimating to a new locale. By consuming local pollen and honey, one's allergies to new flora and fauna can be diminished. Honey and pollen nourish the immune system as well as moderate autoimmune activity. "Modern scientific research has found bee pollen to contain properties beneficial to healing, revitalizing, and protecting against radiation therapy." (Tenney). Also, the pollen will add a little "crunch" to your yogurt, and the honey will add a "creamy" soft texture to your cakes, pies, and cookies. When it comes to baking, it's fun to see how their flavor and texture enhance a favorite recipe.

Black Cohosh (Cimifuga racemosa) rhizomes and roots, native to the Northeastern part of North America. Virtues: adaptogen, alterative, antispasmodic, cardiac adaptogen, diuretic, emmenagogue, nervine, sedative, oxytocic. While the Native Americans nicknamed black cohosh "rattlesnake root" or "snakeroot," since it was useful for snake bites, modern usage focuses on the panoply of female issues black cohosh excels at helping: premenstrual tension, menstrual symptoms, menopausal symptoms, uterine cramps, estrogen deficiency, water retention. It's known to be especially helpful in normalizing the menopause transition. The natural estrogen in black cohosh can hinder the growth of prostate tumors in men. An excellent tonic for the central nervous system, it benefits rheumatism, coughs, lung issues, whooping cough. "Tonic, nervine, anti-spasmodic. Has acquired no little reputation in the treatment of chorea, convulsions, nervous excitability, asthma, and other spasmodic diseases; also in remittent and intermittent fevers, and in acute and chronic rheumatism; is a valuable uterine tonic, and useful in headaches attendant on uterine derangement." (Parke, Davis & Co.) **DO NOT USE DURING PREGNANCY.**

Black Haw (Viburnum prunifolium) dried bark of root and stem, native to North America. Virtues: Anti-spasmodic, sedative, hypotensive, astringent. Excellent for "quieting" uterus cramps and dysmenorrhea; a powerful relaxant for a stressed female system, facilitates uterine relaxation, and a history of being valuable for preventing miscarriage. (Gladstar) Plentiful in steroidal saponins which act as precursors for hormone production by the liver, these can also ease the transition of menopause. Sometimes used as an anti-spasmodic when treating asthma.

Black Walnut (Juglans nigra) hulls and leaves, native to Central and Eastern North America. Virtues: alterative, anthelmintic, anti-galactagogue, antineoplastic, antiseptic, astringent, vulnerary. Useful for the elimination of parasites, tapeworms, and bad bacteria as it oxygenates the blood. The extract has a role in clearing poison oak, ringworm, and skin problems. "…promotes the healing of indolent ulcers, specific and non-specific." (Parke-Davis) It also supports the elimination of toxins and fatty materials as well as balancing sugar levels. Uniquely, it's been noted to restore tooth enamel. And the nuts are a great source of the mood-relaxing serotonin. (As the saying goes, a black walnut is a tough nut to crack. Get yourself an industrial-strength nutcracker—really!)

Blessed Thistle (Cnicus benedictus) entire herb, native the Mediterranean. Virtues: alterative, antibacterial, bitter, blood purifier, emmenagogue, galactagogue. While used traditionally in Europe for smallpox and gangrene, it's associated with digestive problems, stomach, spleen, intestines, gastric disorders, heart problems, poor blood circulation, gallbladder, blood impurities, water retention, liver congestion and repair, and fighting headaches. An amplifier of lactation flow, it can add additional nutrients to mother's milk. On a spiritual level, Blessed Thistle is known for its hardiness and endurance; surely the courage of motherhood warrants this consideration. A must for your morning smoothie.

Blue Cohosh (Caulophyllum thalictrocides) roots, Native to the Northeast in North America. Virtues: alterative, anthelmintic, antispasmodic, diaphoretic, diuretic, emmenagogue, estrogenic, expectorant, oxytocic. The very first medicinal herb I ever took, which worked wonderfully to correct my dysmenorrhea, stimulating my delayed menses. Since it has emmenagogic properties, blue cohosh should **not be used by pregnant women** (yet is an old Native American favorite to ease childbirth). Used to regulate menstrual flow, it has antibacterial properties and a strong antispasmodic effect. Relieves muscle cramps and spasms, inflammation, high blood pressure, and palpitations of the heart. **DO NOT USE DURING PREGNANCY.**

Boneset (Eupatorium perfoliatum) aerial parts, native to North America. Virtues: alterative, anti-inflammatory, antiperiodic, antiviral, diaphoretic, febrifuge, (gentle) purgative, nervine. Probably the first herb introduced to the Mayflower passengers who landed in 1620 on Plymouth Rock, it helped those who'd contracted dengue fever. Taken ill after sailing across the Atlantic, 50 of the 102 passengers wound up with "breakbone fever" and died their first winter in the New World. Dengue fever was called "breakbone fever" in those days because contracting the illness was so painful, it felt like "one's bones were breaking." The Native Americans brought the newcomers this tea, excellent for quelling this influenza, and they recovered. The landed Pilgrims called it "boneset," since they felt their "bones had been set back into place." Research has shown that as a diaphoretic, the sweat glands are stimulated. It activates the kidneys, thereby stimulating the release of toxins. Boneset strengthens the immune system. Coughs, chills, fever, colds, flu, sore throat, and bronchitis pneumonia.

Burdock (Arctium lappa) roots and rhizome, native to Europe. Virtues: Alterative, antineoplastic, antirheumatic, blood purifier, demulcent, diaphoretic, diuretic, vulnerary. For a real rite of passage as an herbalist, go dig up your first burdock. (My first dig, wildcrafting on a mountain, took over an hour.) An alterative, this is a blood cleanser par excellence and has a special affinity for the skin. Carefully carried across the pond by pilgriming goodwives to ensure continued health in the New World, it is now found in meadows and woodlands throughout North America, from Quebec to Alabama. The roots are served as vegetables in Japan, and even Native Americans adopted this broad-leafed plant for skin ailments. Burdock addresses acne, arthritis, colds, eczema, fevers, measles, allergies, kidney problems, skin disorders, tumors, and wounds. Dr. James Duke, a scientist who worked for over 30 years researching the medicinal use of herbs for the Department of Agriculture, states, "Fresh burdock roots contain phytochemicals called polyacetylenes, which can destroy certain bacteria and fungi, (which) perhaps explains the traditional use of this herb as treatment for ringworm, urinary tract infections, and other bacterial onslaughts." A student told me that as a little girl in Sicily, she'd go gathering on the hillsides with her grandmother for tender, springtime burdock leaves. At home, they'd make a tasty side dish of burdock leaves smothered in butter and garlic.

Cardamom (Elettaria cardamomum) seeds, native to India. Virtues: Because it contains the phytochemical cineole, it's a strong antiseptic that kills the bacteria responsible for bad breath. (Duke) A helpful carminative, spleen and stomach tonic, used for infections, liver problems, sore throats. A warm and grateful aromatic, it's found in many, delicious holiday recipes. A little goes a long way in baking; it has a wonderful way of becoming the third or fourth flavor tasted when drinking a blended herbal tea.

Cascara Sagrada (Rhamnus purshiana) bark, North America. Virtues: alterative, anthelmintic, antineoplastic, antispasmodic, hepatic, laxative, lithotripsic, purgative. Named "sacred bark" by the early Spanish explorers probably hints about their convalescence during travels and a testimony to its importance; this herb is an effective intestinal cleanser. It can restore intestinal tone for the peristaltic action to move chyme along. Valuable for treating hemorrhoids due to poor bowel function, it reinforces secretions of the stomach, liver, and pancreas. Helpful in ridding the body of gallstones and worms. Under the categories of prudence and forethought: use only in small doses for a short period of time, not for continuous use. "…[Cascara sagrada] has been aptly called a 'Tonic Laxative,' because of its physiologic action, which seems to be directed to the vaso-motor system, thereby stimulating the secretory apparatus of the alimentary canal and increasing peristaltic action, restoring to normal activity…neither does it, as a rule, cause griping or other unpleasant symptoms." (Parke-Davis)

Catnip (Nepeta cataria) leaves, native to Europe and now in North America. Virtues: antispasmodic, diaphoretic, insomnia, soothing to a colicky infant, can allay gas or painful menstruation, and makes your kitty purr! The oils, which nature intended to act as a bug repellant, can turn big cats into little kittens. (No worries if your cat is one of the handful who doesn't respond.) A gentle, nighttime tea. Most kitties in your neighborhood will enjoy sleeping in your catnip all summer long…

Chamomile (Matricaria chamomilla, Anthemis nobile, and related species) flower, native to Europe and Mediterranean regions. Virtues: anti-inflammatory, antibacterial, antifungal, antiseptic, antispasmodic, emmenagogue, and gentle nervine. While the ancient Egyptians and Romans used chamomile for ague, malaria, and indigestion, Peter Rabbit's mother rightly served him chamomile tea to settle his stomach because he ate too many cabbages. His mother's tea also quieted him down after Mr. McGregor chased Peter out of his garden. Little bunnies and busy urbanites each can sip a relaxing cup of this pretty yellow tea. It plays a supportive role in bedsores, bruises, burns, coughing, digestion, fevers, frostbite, gallbladder problems, gas, insomnia, sore throat, bunions, flu, gouts, infection, motion sickness, stress, wounds, and especially to allay inflammation. This trustworthy flower is also useful for small babies and children suffering from colds, stomach trouble, or colitis. Rosemary Gladstar says, "Chamomile is an excellent healing agent in douche formulas and sitz baths and is used frequently for this purpose in commercial preparations." It combines well with rose hips and stevia for a calming, good-night tea. And, ever versatile, it can be used by blondes to highlight their hair!

Chaparral (Larrea tridentata) leaves and stem, native to the southwestern deserts of the United States. Virtues: Alterative, anodyne, expectorant, parasiticide, a potent healer and cleanser for kidney and bladder infections.

For people who work with chemicals, metal, or aromatic hydrocarbons such as solvents, it is associated with cancer prevention, especially in cases where there's a family history of it. Numerous individuals have claimed success in treating cancer from the use of chaparral. (Tenney) When combined with red root and echinacea, it can help reduce the size of tumors. It has a "dry" taste as a tea. **DO NOT USE DURING PREGNANCY.**

Chasteberry (Vitex angus castus) fruit and berries, native to Mediterranean region and Asia. Virtues: astringent, emmenagogue, normalizes the female system. This deciduous shrub-tree earned its name because the berries are reputed to defuse sexual desire. "(Chasteberry's) normalizing and balancing action is particularly beneficial in treating painful and irregular menstruation, infertility, PMS, menopausal problems, and other hormonal imbalances. It has been found helpful in the treatment of endometriosis and is also useful in normalizing the system after discontinuing birth control pills. Because it stimulates the production of prolactin, vitex is often given to nursing mothers to help ensure a healthy supply of milk." (Gladstar) Painful and irregular menstruation, infertility, clots, cramps, chills, excessive bleeding, scanty bleeding, mood swings, food cravings, depression, and vaginal dryness—a list of complaints Western women have related to their menstrual cycles, which Mother Nature *did not intend* for women to experience. In places where people still live close to nature, the rain forests of South America, the bush in Africa, and the high mountaintops of Asia, women hardly experience these female issues to the degree and frequency of Western women. These other women live within the cycles of nature, with pure food, close community, and an earth spirit theology that affords them good health and grounding. Yet the quick fix techno-brews and relentless drumbeat of urbane, big-city high life, reinforced by social media, disunite people from an earth spirit connection. It shows up in women's menstrual cycles first. One woman I worked with got a cold right before her period; another slept for ten hours two days before her cycle began; and one other woman would get an abscess the size of her fist on her inner thigh each month concurrently with her menses. And how many women have been chided for being in a dark mood "at that time of the month?" As new millennia metropolitan lives are inundated with greater overloads of pollutants, mental strain, and spiritual disharmony, women's cycles are trumpeting to city dwellers, and women in particular, that a modern lifestyle isn't working. I find that a woman's cycle is a "loud" barometer of these boundary breaks. Luckily, chasteberry can also be applied to men's hormonal imbalances, including overactive libido and hormonally induced acne. It really does "level" those sex hormones.

Chickweed (Stellaria media) aerial parts, native to Europe Virtues: alterative, anorectic, blood purifier, demulcent, diuretic, emollient, febrifuge, mucilant, nutritive, pectoral, stomachic. Growing abundantly now in town and country all over North America and even the Artic, chickweed's tender spring leaves are like spinach for your spring salad. Folk uses: valuable for treating blood toxicity, bronchitis, pleurisy, hoarseness, weakness of the bowels, rheumatism, and any form of inflammation. It helps dissolve plaque in blood vessels and other fatty substances. When one of my cats turned 15 years old and began slowing down, chickweed suddenly appeared in my garden next to the weeping cherry tree she liked to sleep under. She nibbled on it daily, and within two weeks, she was curious, up and ready to go on squirrel patrol. I call that good karma.

Cinnamon (Cinnamon zeylanicum, C. aromaticum, C. verum) inner bark, native to Asia. Virtues: alterative, antibacterial, antifungal, antiseptic, astringent, carminative, circulatory stimulant, diaphoretic, emmenagogue, febrifuge, stimulant, stomachic. Employed by the ancient Egyptians, this herbal spice has been in use continuously for several thousand years. Indicated in exhaustion, especially following infections such as the flu, it

allays nausea, checks vomiting, eases allergies, relieves flatulence, indigestion, gastric disorders, bloating, and stimulates the heart. It is used in
Ayurveda herbalism to support normal brain function and a normally, func-
tioning, female reproductive system. The 1865 United States Dispensatory
states, "The U.S. Pharmacopoeia embraces, under the title of cinnamon,
not only bark of that name obtained from island of Ceylon, which is the
only variety recognized in the new British Pharmacopoeia, but also the
commercial cassia, which is imported from China…Indeed, the barks of all
the species of the genus Cinnamomum, possessing analogous properties,
are as much entitled to the common name of cinnamon…" In Ayurvedic
herbalism, cinnamon is a pita herb, increases heat, and cinnamon, like
ginger, nutmeg, cloves, nutmeg, and cardamom, has found its delicious
way into many winter holiday recipes.

Cleavers (Galium aparine) dried aerial parts, native to North America
and Eurasia. Virtues: alterative, anti-inflammatory, aperient, diuretic,
tonic; a superior lymphatic tonic and remedy for kidney and bladder
troubles. Rejuvenating the lymphatic system induces sweeping benefits
to many actions in the body: urinary problems, tumors, jaundice, ulcers,
and internally for wound healing. Folk uses: swollen glands, cancer, nerve
problems. An all-around, daily tonic tea: cleavers and nettles.

Cloves (Eugenia caryophyllata) seeds and flower buds, native to
Indonesia. Virtues: alterative, analgesic, anodyne, anthelmintic, antibacterial, antifungal, antiseptic, aromatic, carminative, circulatory stimulant.
Carried in remedy chests when the Bible was written, cloves were first
introduced to Europe by the Arabians and soon became a favorite on the
spice route from Europe to Asia. The best stimulant of all the aromatics, it
acts as a powerful germicidal agent. One of the oldest remedy recipes: put
a whole clove on an aching tooth. It generates circulation, promotes digestion, allays nausea, and is tasty. No wonder it's always a favorite in baking.

Coltsfoot (Tussilago farfara) flowers and leaves, native to Europe. Virtues: alterative, anti-inflammatory, antitussive, astringent, bitter, demulcent, diaphoretic, diuretic, emollient, expectorant, mucilant, pectoral. Used by the Greeks, Romans, and Chinese for lung conditions, including coughs, asthma, bronchitis, because it soothes the brain's cough-activating mechanism. For a sore throat and excessive mucus, coltsfoot remedies the lungs whether from a cold or cigarette smoking. Named for its leaf shape that resembles a colt's footprint, it was drunk as a tea as well as smoked by the Colonials. The leaf was sometimes employed as a plate when a day in the woods was spent foraging and grazing. "A domestic remedy for coughs and colds…throat pastilles. A valuable combination of coltsfoot, licorice, sugar…horehound, wild cherry, anise…" (Parke Davis)

Comfrey (Symphytum officinale) entire plant, native to Northeast North America. Virtues: demulcent, astringent, and tonic. From Culpepper to the U. S. Pharmacopeia to Dr. James Duke and Rosemary Gladstar, authoritative sources have praised comfrey for its mucilaginous applications to healing internal and external wounds, fractures, sores, and ulcers. It's also valued for bloody urine, stomach, and bowel conditions. One hospital in New York City used to send home new mothers who'd just given birth with a comfrey mixture tea for healing the birth canal. "A syrup made thereof is very effectual for all those inward griefs and hurts…." (Culpepper) When hit by a motorcycle, Rosemary Gladstar writes about taking recovery matters into her own hands and drinking "copious amounts of comfrey [tea]…" Useful too as a salve, it was the first one I made for Molly, the porcupine, who lived at Bear Mountain Zoo. The zookeeper came to my shop and said Molly had a mysterious rash on her tummy. That night, I cut comfrey leaves from my garden, added them to grapeseed oil with calendula, and made six jars of healing salve for Molly. (When it's for an animal, part of the equation includes the animal trying to lick it off; therefore it must be safe internally.) The zookeeper came back the next day, got the salve, and called me four days later to order more jars. As with a number of herbs recently, comfrey has been dissected and parsed by orthodox medicine. Dr. James Duke stated, "Not for long-term internal consumption—in reasonable dosages, no longer than a total of four to six weeks in a year; consult a qualified physician ...comfrey contains pyrrolizidine alkaloids [Pas], which in excessive amounts have been linked to severe, even lethal, liver toxicity. The warnings have given comfrey a bad rap, and even herbalists are divided on whether to use the age-old herb. Some say that is should be applied only externally; others point to research asserting that a cup of comfrey tea possesses less cancer-causing potential than a can of beer."

Cornsilk (Zea mays) strings inside the cornhusk, native to North and South America. Virtues: anodyne, diuretic, demulcent, nephritic. For kidney, bladder, urination problems, and prostate-urination complaints. Salvage the yellow silk of the non-GMO corn, and let it dry out. The cornsilk from the South American purple kculli corn is especially loaded with antioxidants and acts as a hepatic. It can be tinctured or used in salads. "This herb is especially useful for conditions of purulent (pus-forming) decomposition of urine in the bladder. It will cleanse the bladder membranes in cystic catarrh and will manifest antiseptic action when in the presence of morbid deposits." (Green) Cornsilk combines well with saw palmetto and yarrow for prostatitis or enlarged prostate gland. Make the tea, fill a thermos, and sip it all day. "Poco a poco/little by little" is an effective treatment plan.

Damiana (Turnera aphrodisiaca) leaves, native to Central and South America. Virtues: Ancient Mayans used damiana as an aphrodisiac, and Mother Nature has always favored enticing a low libido (rites of spring...). Traditional applications include nervousness, weakness, exhaustion, depression. "Damiana helps to revitalize the body when in a state of exhaustion...and strengthens the nerves and brain." (Tenney) It can be useful in anxiety or depression that may have a sexual factor. "It is a general tonic to the intestines and likewise to the nervous system." (Parke-Davis) Activates the treatment of impotence, it may bring to bear a strengthening of the male system. (Green) It can serve as an unofficial test kit: if someone isn't aroused with damiana's regular use, it can indicate a body too overloaded with anxiety.

Dandelion (Taraxacum officinale) roots, leaves, and the flowers make a tasty, Italian wine, native to Europe. Virtues: revered by the Pilgrims as an alterative, powerful diuretic, cholagogue, anti-rheumatic, and tonic, dandelion came over on the Mayflower. Unlike conventional diuretics, it does not leach potassium from the body and is loaded with potassium itself. Dandelion can revivify the gall bladder and is used as a stimulant in chronic, functional derangement of the liver. Dr. James Duke reminds us, "In French, dandelion is 'pissenlit,' which translates as 'piss in bed,' a rather vulgar reference to the urinary encouragement of this perennial herb." Its early spring leaves are tasty in salads. Dandelion and milk thistle combine well when recovering from alcohol or drug use and may be used long term.

Devil's Claw (Harpagophytum procumbens) rhizome and roots, native to Africa. Virtues: alterative, anodyne, anti-inflammatory, antilithic, anti-rheumatic, blood purifier, diuretic, hepatic, stimulant. Medical research confirms that this rhizome quells inflammation and eases arthritis, body aches, and any inflammatory condition be it acute, adhesive, fibrinous, bacterial, or reactive. Helpful with liver, gallbladder, kidneys, and effects of pollution. Assists in the release of toxic build up in the joints. I was diagnosed with rheumatoid arthritis in 1998. I have never taken one drug on one day for it. I do watch my diet, and if I'm stressed and feeling discomfort, devil's claw is my go-to.

Dong Quai (Angelica sinensis) root, native to China. Virtues: alterative, antibacterial, antineoplastic, antispasmodic, aperient, blood purifier, estrogenic, hypotensive, immunostimulant, sedative. In Traditional Chinese Medicine (TCM), Dong Quai is valued as the queen of female herbs. A blood purifier, it promotes relief for menopause disorders and PMS. Dong quai helps tone and fortify the uterus in preparation for conception. The phytochemicals can activate the production of white blood cells, thereby strengthening the immune system, in turn helping preparation for pregnancy. Additional research suggests that Dong Quai can aid the liver in eliminating toxins, which improves the metabolism of protein. **DO NOT USE DURING PREGNANCY.**

Echinacea (Echinacea angustifolia, Echinacea purpurea, Brauneria angustifolia) root, native to North America. Virtues: adaptogen, alterative, antibiotic, antimicrobial, antineoplastic, antiseptic, antiviral, blood purifier, demulcent, digestive, vulnerary. This garden belle generously used by Native Americans, stimulates the immune response, increases the production of white blood cells, and improves the body's ability to resist infections. Echinacea elevates lymphatic filtration and drainage for removing toxins from the blood. It supports the body's own response to "abscesses, acne, allergies, blood poisoning, boils, cancer, canker sores, carbuncles, chemotherapy, colon cancer, cystitis, dandruff, dental inflammation, dysentery, earache, eczema, gallbladder problems, goiter, gonorrhea, gum disease, headache, herpes, liver cancer, lymph gland enlargement or disease, meningitis, parasitic infections, psoriasis, scarlet fever, sinus problems, skin inflammation, sore throat, tonsillitis, toothache, tuberculosis, varicose veins, whooping cough, yeast infections." (Duke) An excellent blood cleanser, morbid matter is removed via the blood system. Simply, it can shorten the duration of a cold or flu. I agree with Dr. Duke: If someone does have an auto-immune disease, it may be better to try Echinacea in smaller doses, or to use other herbs. One of the prettiest herbs, this pink coneflower heralds the warm months while dressing up your garden.

Elecampane (Inula helenium) root, native to Europe and Northern Asia. Virtues: alterative, antiasthmatic, antibacterial, anticatarrhal, antiseptic, astringent, diaphoretic, diuretic, expectorant, a tonic to mucous membranes. This soothing result applies to lungs and to hemorrhoids. Elecampane has an antibacterial effect which stimulates recovery from chest congestion, coughing, bronchitis, and asthma. Clinical research has found that it contains a powerful antiseptic and bactericide that are efficacious against tuberculosis. Traditionally used to help heal skin infections in horses and sheep, its essential oil has been employed as an anti-inflammatory and antiseptic, especially against bacteria, fungi, and candida. In a wintertime episode of sneezing-coughing-fever-no-sleep, you can begin with elecampane. Definitely time for this nourishing remedy in a good root soup.

Ephedra/Ma Huang (Ephedra sinensis) leaf, native to Asia. Virtues: Anorectic, anticatarrhal, astringent, decongestant, diaphoretic, expectorant, stimulant. Ephedra has been used by Chinese apothecaries for thousands of years to treat acute respiratory problems: asthma, bronchitis, pneumonia, fever, and colds. It's a stimulant, associated with depression and low energy. Germany's Commission E (similar to America's Food and Drug Administration) approves of ephedra: "Diseases of the respiratory tract with mild bronchospasms in adults and children over the age of six." Traditional practitioners still use the herb sparingly for short-term breathing issues. Today's herbalists act with discretion about using it if one is prone to high blood pressure. Recent reports about ephedra make it a case study in the misuse of an ancient remedy. What happened to this esteemed Asian herb has become a cautionary tale for American marketers as well as the health food industry. Twenty-first century snake oil salesman pitched an extract of this herb, *ephedrine*, for weight loss and sustained energy. Steve Belcher of the Orioles, age 23, died in 2003, and "A dietary supplement with ephedra was linked to Bechler's death. He had collapsed during practice Sunday and had been taken to the hospital by ambulance." (HistoricBaseball.com) Many newspapers repeated this narrative without distinguishing the difference between the whole herb, *ephedra,* and a megadose of the extract, *ephedrine.* Medically, it was reported he died from heat stroke playing baseball in the hot Florida sun while taking weight loss supplements. Mark Blumenthal of the American Botanical Council did my radio show, The Urban Herbalist, for one hour within the week of Bechler's death, and we went back and forth, particularizing the differences between extracts and the complete nutritional matrix of the plant, as well as the detailed, clinical and empiric evidence of several thousand years, which positively illustrated the efficacy of this herb. The idea was to educate the public about the differences between a plant and a product. A tragedy to lose this up-and-coming athlete, the mainstream media kept pressing on the herbal connection; modern day herbalists were up against modern day corporations. Dr. James Duke stated, "Ephedra is, essentially, prescription medication. Pseudoephedrine [from ephedra] is the active ingredient in Sudafed and other decongestants. Ephedrine hydrochloride is commonly found not only in health food stores but at truck stops in various parts of the country…a handful of people have died over the past few years from abusing ephedra products, prompting the FDA to issue warnings against their use and to consider banning the substance entirely…" When I interviewed a Chinese doctor about ephedra, the first thing he said was, "But you are only supposed to take it for a short period of time." This raises quite an issue for doctors, midwives, apothecaries, shamen, wise women, apprentices, and interns to be debated ad nauseum. A substance, a plant, that, when used correctly, can be effective in health care—so how do you get people *to use it correctly?* (When I still got allergies, I used to drink Ma huang tea daily during the hay fever season, one cup every morning, for about two weeks. See the American Botanical Council article on the current ban of ephedra.)

False Unicorn Root (Charmelirium luteum) roots, native to Eastern North America. Virtues: alterative (stimulating), anthelmintic, aphrodisiac, diuretic, emetic (large doses), estrogenic, stimulates and strengthens the reproductive organs in both men and women. It encourages fertility, especially in women, and is sometimes an ally for menopause. Native American women regularly nibbled the roots to maintain their beneficial effects for their reproductive systems, and Eclectic doctors recommended false unicorn root for both men and women to promote fertility. It can restore uterine tone, be applied to Bright's disease, and treat headaches (commonly due to hormonal imbalance). **DO NOT USE DURING PREGNANCY.**

Fennel (Foeniculum valgare) seeds, native to southern Europe and Asia Minor. Virtues: appetite suppressant; carminative—good stomach and intestinal remedy; helps in flow of mother's milk. Fennel also combines well with other bitter herbs blended for a tea or culinary mixture.

Fenugreek (Trigonella foenum-graecum) seeds, native to Mediterranean. Virtues: alterative, anticatarrhal, anti-inflammatory, antiseptic, aphrodisiac, bitter, demulcent, emollient, expectorant, galactagogue. An acclaimed cooking spice, fenugreek has the ability to soften and dissolve hardened masses of accumulated mucus, hasten apoptosis, and expel toxic waste through the lymphatic system. Likewise, ancient Egypt, Greece, and Rome considered it a panacea for bronchial issues, tuberculosis, and skin problems.

Feverfew (Tanacetum parthenium and Chrysanthemum parthenium) leaves, native to southeastern Europe. Virtues: alterative, analgesic, anti-inflammatory, antimicrobial, aromatic, bitter, carminative, emmenagogue, febrifuge, nervine, parasiticide, mild purgative, vasodilator. Oh those aching pains! Revered in ancient Greece, feverfew has a deserved reputation for modulating migraines and easing inflammation, aches, dizziness, chills, fever, indigestion, tinnitus, and worms. Furthermore, it helps with morphine addiction and opium addiction. This is a good herb to work with "poco a poco, little by little" daily, to assist with homeostasis. It's often employed in flatulent or atonic dyspepsia.

Cannabidiol (CBD) is a compound found in marijuana (Cannabis indica and Cannabis sativa) leaves, native to Central Asia. CBD can be derived from hemp or from non-hemp plants. Hemp is defined as any part of the cannabis sativa plant with no more than 0.3% of tetrahydrocannabinol (THC), the mind-altering substance in marijuana. (cdc.gov)

Cannabis Sativia "Narcotic, producing in full doses exhilaration, intoxication and delirious hallucinations. Recommended in delirium tremens, certain forms of insanity, delirium after fever, softening of the brain and conditions involving anemia of the cortex, to check excessive or painful cough, to relieve migraine, to allay itching of eczema, to prevent the griping of certain cathartics, etc." (Parke-Davis 1901)

Cannabis indica (Indian Hemp), Cannabis sativa (Indian Hemp), Cannabis americana (American Cannabis)
"In large doses it causes a peculiar but generally pleasant form of intoxication, during which the particular traits of the individual are exaggerated, and the ideas follow each other so rapidly as to produce a sense of great prolongation of time..." (Therapeutics Materia Medica and Pharmacy 1912)
    "Extract of hemp is a powerful narcotic, causing exhilaration, intoxication, delirious hallucinations, and, in its subsequent action, drowsiness and stupor, with little effect upon the circulation. It is asserted also to act as a decided aphrodisiac, to increase the appetite..." (United States Dispensatory 1861)

"In the stage of intoxication persons under its influence become much more excited than do the devotees of alcohol...It is used to relieve spasm and dull pain, especially in neuralgia, migraine, asthma, colic, and pain originating in the ovaries or womb. It is also given for sleepless-ness..." (Health Knowledge 1927)

The cache of smoking marijuana (or the medicinal use of a canna-bis tincture) is well documented in medical texts as well as spritely folk lore. Some unacquainted bystanders today believe that if one ingests the rising star "CBD oil," openly peddled in the marketplace today, then a person can get some kind of "high." Not so. A rigorous manufacturing procedure extracts the cannabidiol, one of over 400 chemicals found in cannabis, concentrates the extract, and refines its bioavailability for sale as an anti-depressant or pain reliever. As recreational marijuana is being legalized across the United States, the intensity of Mother Nature's nascent, sticky bush has been magnified a hundred-fold. The results of CBD oil and dispensary marijuana are two separate categories. The inherent, endocan-nabinoid system in humans consists of cannabinoid receptors, endogenous cannabinoids, and our own enzymes, which interact together, allowing the system to function. "Migraine, fibromyalgia, IBS, and related conditions display common clinical, biochemical, and pathophysiological patterns that suggest an underlying endocannabinoid deficiency." (www.cbdmd. com) It is best to not double up, i.e., to use another anodyne or intoxicant while ingesting cannabis or CBD oil. As the FDA scrambles to investigate and legislate this marketplace, it's worth noting that *individual results will vary...*

Garcinia (Garcinia cambogia) fruit, native to Asia and Australia. Virtues: Anorectic, anticatarrhal, aperient, thermogenetic, stimulant. When the health issue is obesity, you can begin with garcinia. An overnight star thanks to Dr. Oz's recommendation, this little fruit has generated seminars at health food industry conventions about the "Dr. Oz effect." Weight loss is always one of the top five health issues people ask about when turning to alternative health. *Providing someone exercises and eats a healthy diet,* garcinia can speed up weight-loss. It's been shown to curb appetite, burn fat, and slow down the accumulation of adipose tissue around the waist.

Garlic (Allium sativum) bulb, native to Middle Asia. Virtues: Adaptogen, alterative, antibiotic, anticoagulant, antifungal, antineoplastic, antiseptic, blood purifier, diaphoretic, digestive, expectorant, febrifuge, rubefacient, stimulant, vulnerary. *What doesn't taste good smothered in garlic and butter?* Called "the poor man's penicillin," this anti-viral is largely used for infections of the respiratory system. It can activate the lymphatic system to rid the body of toxins. It will support the development of natural, intestinal bacteria while killing pathogenic organisms. Empiric records as well as scientific research have catalogued the numerous ailments and conditions garlic addresses. A must for your healing cupboard.

Ginger (Zingiber officinale) rhizome/root, native to Southeast Asia. Virtues: Alterative, antacid, anti-inflammatory, carminative, diaphoretic, diuretic, febrifuge, sialagogue, stimulant. Chinese apothecaries and the celebrated Greek historian Dioscorides each recommended ginger for digestive issues including the production of gastric juices. Agreeably, it quells nausea and motion sickness. It's a favorite of wise women for uterine cramps and morning sickness. Given that ginger is a pita herb in Ayurveda, it's not surprising that, like other pita herbs—cinnamon and cardamon—ginger is favored for winter-holiday recipes: ginger-bread men, ginger-spiced cakes, cinnamon and ginger in oatmeal, hot chocolate with ginger. (As I blend teas and create recipes, ginger can go just about anywhere.)

Ginseng (Panax ginseng, native to Asia; Panax quinquefolius, [American Ginseng] native to North America) root. Virtues: adaptogen, alterative, anti-depressive, stimulant, stomachic, a physical and mental performance tonic. Prescribed steadily in Asia for thousands of years, sold widely around the world as a rejuvenator, and revered for its restoration of vitality, this herb has traditional and scientific credits to its name. Interestingly, the Asian market venerates Panax quinquefolius so highly, it was one of the cash crops that saved the fledgling United States of America from going bankrupt after the Revolutionary War. Uplifts depression, reduces high blood pressure, elevates low blood pressure, activates memory and attention, and invigorates the immune system. Because it's been touted for its strong tonic qualities, ginseng is frequently, scientifically tested for its credentials. There's an Asian apothecary in New York which only sells various species of ginseng, and customers travel there from up and down the Eastern seaboard. Extensively prescribed in Traditional Chinese medicine for stamina, it's best not to combine it with other stimulants.

Ginkgo (Gingko biloba) leaves, native to China. Virtues: adaptogen, alterative, antioxidant, antiseptic, stimulant. Before the Tyrannosaurus Rex and the Stegosaurus started leaving big footprints and extravagant fossils on seven continents, the ginkgo tree was well-established. History has accorded it the title of "living fossil," and one tree can last over 1,000 years. Brought from China back to England, one tree planted in 1762 still grows in Kew Gardens, London. A deciduous tree, the Chinese began using ginkgo several thousand years ago to hold in abeyance age-related mental decline. Happily, science and research caught up with arcane herbology and conducted clinical trials on the efficacy of this singular herb. Ginkgo boosts the brain function for different applications: Alzheimer's disease, attention span, dementia, memory, senility, mental focus. Additionally, it helps prevent strokes by preventing the formation of blood clots, increases oxygen to the brain, and quells inflammation. It aids multiple sclerosis, stress, ADD, muscular degeneration, mood swings, depression, migraines, arthritis, angina, altitude sickness, menstrual irregularities, PMS, and

Raynaud's disease. Delightfully, certain New York City tourist books single out city blocks with older ginkgo trees because their foliage is both decorative and unique. In New York, that's saying something.

Goat's Rue (Galega officinalis) dried aerial parts, native to Middle East and Southern Europe. Virtues: bitter, diuretic, diaphoretic, galactagogue, hypoglycemic. Shepherds in the Alps noticed when goats got pregnant, they started munching on this perennial shrub. The mama goats always had plenty of milk. While traditionally having played a role in fevers, the plague, and worms, its two, time-honored virtues have been to enhance lactation for new mothers and to balance blood sugar. It aids the pancreas for a diabetic.

Goldenseal (Hydrastis canadensis) root, native to North America. Virtues: adaptogen, alterative, anthelmintic, antibiotic, antiseptic, chol-agogue, emmenagogue, hepatic, nephritic, purgative (mild), stomachic, tonic. A Native American favorite, golden seal was one of the first herbs adopted by the early colonists. Goldenseal's wondrous effect on infec-tion-fighting made it a New World commodity sold widely across the globe, thereby helping the fledgling United States avoid bankruptcy after the Revolutionary War. It's been listed in the United States Pharmacopoeia and is still used by drug companies as a source for extracts. Continuous studies find it addresses infections, viruses, colds, inflammation, infections, bronchitis, bladder congestion, ulcers, liver congestion, and increases intestinal secretions and bile flow. Its antibiotic properties are due to the alkaloid content, which includes berberine (found also in Oregon grape root and barberry). Favored by Native Americans as a worthy eyewash, I've decocted a pot of tea, drank some, and then used some on my eyes (let it cool down). Caution: It is best used for short periods of time as it builds up the mucosa of the body. Also, overuse may cause the body "to get used to it" so larger and larger doses will be needed to stimulate body systems.

"Goldenseal should be used during pregnancy with caution. Large doses stimulate involuntary muscles of the uterus and may cause premature contractions." (Gladstar) "[Golden seal] is a most excellent remedy for colds, la grippe, and all kinds of stomach and liver troubles. It exerts a special influence on all the mucous membranes and tissues with which it comes in contact." (Kloss) Also, when you dig up a four-year-old plant, you'll find beautiful, dancing, golden roots!

Green Tea (Camellia sinensis) leaves, native to Asia. Virtues: antioxidant, anti-depressive, anti-inflammatory, antineoplastic, cardiac tonic, stimulant. This fail-safe diuretic, cardio protector, and mood elevator is the world's second-most-often-sipped beverage. Given how easily it grows and is commercially traded, green tea is sometimes overlooked for its real medicinal virtues. It's a useful adjuvant for a daily regimen. From the 1865 U.S. Pharmacopeia: "Tea is astringent and gently excitant…render it capable of very extensive application as a medicine….should be avoided by dyspeptic individuals, and by those whose nervous systems are peculiarly excitable. As a medicine, tea may sometimes be given advantageously in diarrhea (sic) and a strong infusion will often be found to relieve nervous headache…"

Gymnema (Gymnema sylvestre) leaves, native to Asia, Africa, and Australia. Virtues: antiperiodic, diuretic, stomachic, sweetness-taste-blocker. Ayurvedic herbalism has promoted gymnema for 5,000 years, and only recently has it found a place in American health food stores. Modern science confirms what Ayurvedic herbalists have known: gymnema blocks not only the taste of sugar, but also the absorption of sugar by the body. Gymnema opposes a desire for any kind of sweetness. In turn, this stimulates the function of the liver and pancreas. "Supports normal function of the pancreas, normal appetite levels; name means "sugar destroyer" in Hindi; contains no stimulants or thermogenics but supports the proper

absorption of sugar and helps reduce sugar cravings." (Himalaya USA)....
to seriously curb your sweet tooth...

Hawthorn Berries (Crataegus oxyacanthoides) berries, native to North America, Europe, and East Asia. Virtues: alterative, antispasmodic, astringent, cardio alterative, diuretic, sedative, vasodilator. Mother Nature generously planted hawthorn across the globe, so ancient Greeks, Romans, and Chinese all promoted these berries as a cardio and circulatory tonic. Its mild, sedative attribute helps ease stress, insomnia, and high blood pressure in turn alleviating additional consequences for heart health. Between environmental toxins and a high-octane-caffeine-lifestyle, hawthorn comforts many heart conditions. "...hawthorn extracts have a marked impact on angina pectoris (the chest pains caused by dearth of blood to an overtaxed heart), atherosclerosis (the blood-blocking buildup of oxidized cholesterol inside arteries), the artery-constricting pressure of hypertension, and the fluid buildup of congestive heart failure." (Duke) Additionally, the macerated leaves and berries were used as a poultice for removing bramble, thorns, and splinters.

Hops (Humulus lupulus) flower, native to Europe, Southwestern Asia, and North America. Virtues: anaphrodisiac, anodyne, antibacterial, antibiotic, carminative, cholagogue, diuretic, nervine, sedative, stomachic, vulnerary. For the last 9,000 years, malts, ales, and beer have been made with hops. Popular with Vikings, hops hold a special place in bacchanalia across many cultures, but these are the fermented, alcoholic versions of the beverage. Hops tea has been enlisted as a remedy for headaches, indigestion, pains, gastric disorders, hyperactivity, insomnia, anxiety, gas, liver disorders, menstrual discomforts, neuralgia, rheumatism, sleeplessness, and restlessness. Also, it tops the apothecary's list to subdue "excessive sexual desire." A requested need before modern birth control changed the social mores about open sexual activity, hops was employed by armies, the ministry, and midwives to diminish desirous adult behavior. This is still a sought-after need. I remember a young army veteran, just back from Iraq, and readjusting to civilian life here on the East Coast, away from his family roots in the Midwest. For the first time, he was out on his own, in a new state, in a new job, decompressing from the front lines of war, and, in his words, didn't want "to spend Saturday nights in bars hunting women." He wanted a year to find himself. I admired this young man's sensibility and planning. I told him to drink a nice, big cup of hops tea every night about an hour before bedtime. It would help him destress (less PTSD), get enough sleep, and not "spill his seed..."

Juniper Berry (Juniperus communis) berries, native to North America, Europe, Asia, and Africa. Virtues: anodyne, antispasmodic, aromatic, astringent, carminative, diuretic, emmenagogue, litholitic, stimulant. From the ancient Greeks to Culpepper, herbalists have brewed juniper berries. High in natural insulin and excellent for infections, it decreases disorders which cause uric acid to be retained in the body. Enlisted as a urinary tract antiseptic, Juniper berries can assist with bladder disorders, prostate disorders, kidney stones, kidney infections, water retention, adrenal gland problems, rheumatism, ague, insect bites, excess mucus, gleet, gout, and recovery from excessive drug use. Duke reports, "It also contains a powerful virus-killing substance, deoxypodophyllotoxin, and other phytochemicals that can fight herpes and influenza." And Kloss recommended, "Juniper berries are excellent as a spray or fumigation of a room in which there has been a patient with an infectious disease, as it thoroughly destroys all fungi."

Native Americans used crushed sweet-tart juniper berries in cakes for winter survival. Here is a colonial recipe:

"Honey Cake: Sift into a pan a pound of flour, and rub into it three-quarters of a pound of butter; and then mix in a large tea-cup full of brown sugar that has been crushed fine with a rolling-pin; and three table-spoons of ginger. Also, if you choose, add in two table-spoons of caraway seeds. Beat five eggs very light, and stir them into the mixture alternately with a pint of strained honey. Stir the whole very hard; putting in, at the least, a very small-teaspoonful of pearl-ash *[In colonial cooking, before baking powder was invented, pearl-ash was used as leavening. Instead, for this recipe, blend in ½ teaspoon of baking powder and a heaping teaspoon of finely ground juniper berries.]* melted in a little lukewarm water.

Put the mixture into a square pan, well buttered; set it in a moderate oven, and bake it at least an hour. If thick, it must remain longer in the oven. Cut it into squares, when cold. It will keep a week, but is best fresh." (Alice Cooke Brown)

Kelp (Fucus vesiculosus) entire plant, native to the Pacific Coast, from Alaska and Canada to the shores of Baja, California. Virtues: alterative, antibiotic, demulcent, diuretic, hypotensive, nutritive. Kelp sea forests are composed of rapidly growing brown algae, and sea vegetables deeply resonate with the ancient harmonies of human bodies. Sea vegetables are loaded with minerals and nourish the entire endocrine system. Kelp activates the thyroid, stimulates metabolism, increases the rate of metabolism, and in particular, rebalances female hormones (helpful for excessive cycle bleeding). Kelp is associated with adrenal glands, lack of energy, fatigue, infections, headaches, pancreatic problems, tumors, gas, diabetes, acne/skin problems, kidney problems, and prostate problems. I've found it's a wonderful "secret ingredient" for any recipe when adding a tad of salt.

Lady's Mantle (Alchemilla vulgaris) aerial parts, native to Turkey and the Carpathian Mountains. Virtues: Astringent, diuretic, anti-inflammatory, vulnerary. A time-honored "woman's herb," lady's mantle has a unique role in the panoply of women's ailments. It acts as an astringent to excessive bleeding for a woman. This is valuable for young women whose cycles are adjusting, to reducing hemorrhaging after childbirth, to menopause when infrequent menses may extend for days. It's also nourishing after childbirth, improving vitality, and allaying depression. It helps lessen period pains and speeds up healing cuts and wounds. Its lacy leaves and dainty flowers will adorn your garden pathways.

Lavender (Lavandula officinalis) flowers and leaves, native to the Mediterranean. Virtues: carminative, (mild) exhilarant, nervine, stimulant, vulnerary, and calms nausea, flatulent colic, and gastric distress. Rosemary Gladstar calls lavender a crone among herbs, for it's been welcomed into every garden, everywhere it's traveled, and continues bringing healing and happiness. Perhaps the best-known aromatic, it initiated that category when its oil, antiseptic and healing to skin wounds, first scented the tip of a lady's handkerchief. (Never ingest the oil.) Traditionally, it calmed nerves and is still used widely in aromatherapy for depression. Sachets of lavender flowers have been carried, put into drawers, and adorned sacred alters as well as Victorian drawing rooms. A calming tea can be made from the flowers, and for headaches, combine lavender with lemon balm and skullcap. With its exceptionally high concentration of volatile oils, it may be used in baths, simmering pots, and massage oils.

Lemon Balm (Melissa officinalis) leaves, native to Europe. Virtues: antidepressant, antihistamine, antispasmodic, antiviral, anodyne, aromatic, digestants, grounding, hypotensive, nervine, sedative, especially during periods of prolonged stress. During the age of exploration into the New World, it's easy to imagine European royalty sipping their lemon balm tea, confabulating after dinner about a certain explorer who'd neither written lately nor returned with a shipload of gold. Its reputation was so esteemed, it was bequeathed from court to court, notable for its immediate effects. It can quell a headache, depression, and excessive stress with good results.

Noted for helping with spasms in the digestive tract, other therapeutic uses include cold sores, nervousness, stomach disease, heart disease, hysteria, melancholy, menstrual pains, mucous membrane inflammation, and nausea. Rosemary Gladstar recommends it as a good, safe companion herb for pregnant women. It can also combine with nettles during pregnancy for women who suffer from allergies. It adds a nice touch of lemon and greens to any soup. When I was first studying herbs, inhaling my dozen, thick, college textbooks while riding subways four hours daily, writing term papers, and burying my nose in court documents at Brooklyn Supreme Court, it was nice to come home and sip my sweet melissa tea.

Licorice Root (Glycyrrhiza glabra) dried roots, Middle East Origin, used from Rome to China. Virtues: alterative, anti-inflammatory, expectorant, demulcent, emollient, purgative (mild), sialagogue, adrenal support. A playful sweetener and endocrine agent promoting endurance, licorice can nourish the adrenal glands after exhaustion. It counteracts stress. It's a tasty, beneficial tea for coughs, respiratory issues, and other chest complaints. The list of traditional folk uses includes: constipation, boils, earaches, bronchial irritation, eczema, dizziness, healing the intestinal tract (gastric and duodenal ulcers). "The large doses sometimes necessary to generate a therapeutic effect can cause side effects, including high blood pressure, water retention, tissue swelling, weight gain, headache, lethargy, and skewed potassium and sodium levels. The side effects result from increasing levels of cortisol and other adrenal hormones. There is one instance in which the side effects are a welcomed blessing: Addison's disease, in which the adrenal glands don't secrete enough cortisol and aldosterone, leaving you weak and emaciated, among other consequences." (Duke) Licorice is best used throughout the day for short periods of time. Moreover, the next time you're camping, take along whole licorice sticks (dried roots). They're excellent in lieu of a tooth brush, and you get an extra boost hiking up that mountain.

Meadowsweet (Filipendula ulmaria) leaves and flowers, native to North America. Virtues: anodyne, antacid, antiarthritic, antiemetic, anti-inflammatory, astringent, stomachic. This is one of the best-named herbs in the book: a full-blooming meadowsweet bush will perfume an entire pasture. It soothes the mucous membranes of the digestive tract and is good in the treatment of heartburn, hyperactivity, gastritis, peptic ulceration, recovery from diarrhea, indigestion, peptic ulcers, and other intestinal issues. Meadowsweet even contains salicin, found in white willow bark, the original aspirin, helpful for arthritis, muscles, and joints. Furthermore, the flowers lend an almond flavor to smoothies, mead, herbal wines, morning muffins, jams, jellies, and stewed fruits. Lavender, lemon balm, and meadowsweet were favorite strewing herbs for Renaissance hand fastings and weddings.

Milk Thistle (Silybum marianum) seeds, native to Europe. Virtues: Alterative, anti-depressive, antioxidant, demulcent, galactagogue, hepatic, stimulant, supreme liver cleanser. Amongst the many jobs Mother Nature has assigned the liver is the master task of detoxification. Unlike any drug in the marketplace today, the silymarin in milk thistle regenerates liver cells and restores the liver from degradation by pollutants, intoxicant additives, and even excessive viral disrupters. Extensive clinical research shows that silymarin protects the liver from chemical damage. Known for restoring the liver in cases of cirrhosis, hepatitis, environmental pollutants, excessive drug abuse, chemotherapy, and radiation, milk thistle has been a traditional remedy for jaundice, poisoning, depression, fatty deposits, and even menstrual symptoms. "…in modern phytotherapy, the herb is indicated for a whole range of liver and gallbladder conditions, including hepatitis and cirrhosis." (Hoffman) The secondary list of activities for milk thistle are impressive too: speeds up wound healing, restores appetite, promotes better sleep, increases bile secretion, supports immune function. When the body is purified, everything works better. Think about how much more light shines through a room when you wash the windows. "As the name implies, milk thistle promotes milk secretion and is perfectly safe for use by breast-feeding mothers." (Hoffman) The medicinal constituents are not easily decocted; best to grind this one to be used as powder or simply eat it. A must for your herbal cupboard. When I taught college in the biology department, my college class motto was, "Love your liver!"

Moringa (Moringa oleifea) leaves, pods, seeds, native to Asia and Africa. Virtues: antibacterial, antibiotic, antioxidant, anti-inflammatory, antispasmodic, diuretic, galactagogue, hepatoprotective, nervine. This eclectic superfood has been around for centuries in the old world and recently was introduced to North America. Tenacious, resilient, and versatile, it likes hot, rugged growing conditions and offers up in return nourishment, stress reduction, alleviation from inflammation, and help with water treatment. Withstanding drought and poor soils have made moringa an important source of food and medicine in underserved countries. "All parts of the moringa tree—bark, pods, leaves, nuts, seeds, tubers, roots, and flowers— are edible and have been analyzed for their nutrient and phytochemical contents." (Herbalgram) Traditional uses include rheumatism, bronchial asthma, venomous bites, allergies, and malnutrition. "Quercetin, tannins, and saponins also contribute to moringa's leaf's anti-inflammatory and cancer prevention potential." (Herbalgram) "Moringa leaf extracts have been shown to reduce oxidative stress and brain lipid peroxidation in cultured nerve cells while increasing levels of superoxide dismutase and catalase, enzymes with potent antioxidant activity." (Herbalgram) "Moringa seeds have been gaining recognition and use as a natural water treatment in urban and rural areas. Frequently, drinking water must be treated physically and chemically, through coagulation and flocculation processes using chemical coagulants, to make it drinkable. Water is often treated with aluminum sulfate or ferric chloride, but the use of moringa seeds shows promise in completely or partly replacing coagulating agents, reducing cost and improving human and environmental health." (Herbalgram) Perhaps Mother Nature debuted moringa here because its virtues so aptly address our contemporary health challenges.

Motherwort (Leonurus cardiaca) leaves, native to Southeastern Europe and Central Asia. Virtues: antispasmodic, bitter, cardiotonic, cardio depressant, emmenagogue, hepatic, hypotensive, nervine, stomatic. Here is a superior uterine tonic when preparing for motherhood, *not for use during pregnancy*. It's valuable for relieving delayed menses, soothing menstrual cramps, increasing a scanty menstrual flow, and enriching the womb. Likewise, it's valuable as a cardiotonic for heart disease, irregular heart rhythm, high blood pressure, and antispasmodic. It assists in insomnia, rapid heart rate, stroke, anxiety, gas, menstrual pain, sciatica, heart disease, and hyperthyroidism (Graves' disease). A warm poultice of the leaves can help with cramps. In my Preparation for Pregnancy workshops, motherwort is always on the checklist. One woman noted that after taking it, she felt "refreshed" enough to finish the baby's room and joyfully indulged her nesting instincts by shopping for paint colors. **DO NOT USE DURING PREGNANCY**.

Mugwort (Artemisia vulgaris) leaves, native to Europe and parts of Asia and Africa. Virtues: anti-depressant, bitter, carminative, emmenagogue, nervine. Every Renaissance goodwife knew her mothercrafting included making mugwort pillows, a mirific aid in sleeping. Renaissance children flocked to the fields each spring to gather mugwort leaves for stuffing and fluffing household pillow bags. Additionally, a cup of mugwort tea is a relaxing, sleeping tonic and activates the liver and digestion. Science supports its aid in promoting normal menstrual flow, and from Culpepper's Complete Herbal, 1653: "Mugwort is with good success put among other herbs that are boiled for women to apply the hot decoction to draw down their courses, to help the delivery of the birth, and expel the after-birth..." From Parke-Davis, 1901, "Among German practitioners it is esteemed [as] an emmenagogue, and of value in epilepsy and chorea." **DO NOT USE DURING PREGNANCY.**

Mullein (Verbascum thapsus) leaves, native to Europe, Africa, and the Eurasia area. Virtues: analgesic, anti-inflammatory, antispasmodic, antitussive, demulcent, expectorant, mucilant, pectoral, vulnerary. The tea can be used as a gargle, pain killer, to induce sleep, and for calming inflamed and irritated nerves. Works well in controlling coughs, cramps, and spasms while loosening mucus. A six-foot-tall stately plant, mullein's versatile traditional uses include being smoked in Colonial pipes as well as the fluffy leaves being used to line shoes during those cold, Colonial winters. Additional folk uses include crushing the flowers for warts, and making a fomentation for swollen joints, testicles, or scrotum. With dainty, yellow leaves atop its stately stalk, it's a fantastic plant for introducing children to nature. A single mullein can drop a thousand seeds by summer's end. These tiny seedlings can be planted in egg cartons cups to illustrate the growing cycle, another seasonal activity with the kids.

Nettles (Urtica dioica) a.k.a. stinging nettles, aerial parts, native to Europe, Asia, and North Africa. Virtues: Adaptogen, alterative, antiseptic, astringent, blood purifier, diuretic, galactagogue, nutritive, full of minerals. With a record several thousand years old, a stinging nettles stem can be used to urticate one's self for arthritis, rashes, and sciatica. This selected, self-flagellation has a heritage known to bring arthritic relief. Unlike being pricked by a rose, the fuzzy, prickly hairs are much tinier. The relief results from the plant releasing its own chemical, for which the body composes its own chemical response. When infused as a tea, it forfeits its "protector" biochemical compound and becomes a good source of chlorophyll; a cup of nettles tea is like drinking a cup of vitamins. It helps with respiratory infections, asthma, and aids recovery from anemia, low energy, and exhaustion, *all in one plant.*

Nutmeg (Myristica frangrans) the kernel of the ripe seed, native to Indonesia. Virtues: anodyne, astringent, carminative. An aromatic stomatic of agreeable flavor, nutmeg's famous for its wonderful flavor in baking. It promotes digestion, increases appetite, and relieves intestinal spasm and flatulence. Employed as an astringent in diarrheas and dysentery, it's also a stimulant to the nerves, and perks up memory and cognitive function. **DO NOT USE DURING PREGNANCY.**

Oatstraw (Avena sativa) stem, native to the Fertile Crescent—the Eurasia bridge. Virtues: alterative, demulcent, nervine, nutritive, vulnerary. Rich in body-building materials, oatstraw tea was highly recommended by the 19th century Eclectic doctors as a nerve tonic. The silica in oatstraw encourages the excretion of gout-causing uric acid and benefits the brain as well. Antidepressant, insomnia, intestinal disease, stomach disease, urinary tract infections. Traditional: hot compresses of oats relieve pain from kidney stone attacks. The paste/poultice is good for chicken pox. All parts of avena sativa can have a place in your diet: oatstraw as a quieting tea, oatmeal for breakfast and cookies, oat bran to support the intestines. (This is a good one for a hyperactive child.)

Oregano (Origanum majorana, Origanum vulgare) a.k.a., Marjoram, leaf, native to the Mediterranean and Southwest Eurasia. Virtues: anodyne, antiseptic, anticatarrhal, antiseptic, antispasmodic, antiviral, carminative, digestant, diaphoretic, expectorant. While the ancient Greeks showed reverence for oregano with garlands festooning the high ceremonies of weddings and funerals, no American pizza would be complete without it. Older materia medica refer to the common name, marjoram, *origanum majorana*, while the species *origanum vulgare* usually takes the Spanish name, oregano. For Spanish cooking, do use *origanum vulgare*. This popular, culinary herb became a staple for both its flavor and for being so good in fighting off illnesses. Folk uses include: cough, consumption, spleen, to increase urine, insect and snake bites, dropsy, jaundice, toothache, head-ache, gastritis, nausea, seasickness, edema, urinary incontinence, and fungal infections (topical and internal). Conjointly, Spanish, Mexican, noble vegetarian, and soup dishes are bespiced flavorfully with this immune booster. A bonus for your cupboard.

Pau d'arco (Tabebuia, various species) inner bark, native to South America. Virtues: adaptogen, alterative, analgesic, antifungal, antimicrobial, antineoplastic, antiviral, blood purifier. An ancient remedy employed by the Incas, pau d'arco was assigned to fight fungal infections, liver disorders, blood impurities, lung disorders, colitis, constipation, intestinal issues, gastric ulcers, snake bites, arthritis, inflammation of the prostate gland (prostatitis), fevers, dysentery, boils, ulcers, various cancers, and malaria. Used as an anti-tumor remedy and called the "everything herb," it works as an antioxidant and immune system booster. Pau d'arco became a go-to remedy during the Covid-19 pandemic. Consider it to be "auxiliary troops" when your immune system battles with illnesses. It gets in there and fights the good fight for you. **DO NOT USE DURING PREGNANCY.**

Pennyroyal (Hedeoma pulegioides and mentha pulegium labiatae) leaves, native to Europe, North Africa, and Middle East. Virtues: alterative, antispasmodic, antivenomous, aromatic, carminative, decongestant, diaphoretic, diuretic, emmenagogue, nervine, oxytocic, parasiticide, stimulant, stomachic. A member of the mint family, pennyroyal helps regulate a maiden's menses. It treats colds, cramps, irregular menses, flu, headaches, migraines, nausea, phlegm, tuberculosis, vertigo, pleurisy, and bronchitis. Additionally, pennyroyal's nickname during Renaissance times was "fleawort" because it kept fleas away from the garden and house. In my garden, I like planting it next to the catnip since I know the cats will be sleeping there all summer. Furthermore, you can bathe your dog in a light, pennyroyal tea. **DO NOT USE DURING PREGNANCY.**

From Gerard's 1633 Materia Medica: "Pennie Royall, or pudding grasse Pulegium regium vulgatam so is exceedingly well knowne to all our English Nation, that it needeth no description, being our common Pennie Royall....The Vertues.

A. Pennie Royal boyled in wine and drunken, provoketh the monethly termes, bringeth forth the secondine: it provoketh urine, and breatketh the stone, especially of the kidnies.

B. Pennie Royall taken with hony clenseth the lungs, and cleareth the breast from all grosse and thicke humours.

C. The same taken with hony and Aloes, purgeth by stoole melancholy humours, helpeth the crampe and drawing together of sinews.

D. The same taken with water and vinegre asswageth the inordinate desire to vomit, and the paines of the stomacke.

E. If you have when you are at the sea Penny Royall in great quantitie dry, and cast it into corrupt water, it helpeth it much, neither will it hurt them that drinke thereof."

Peppermint (Mentha Piperita) leaves, native to Europe and the Middle East. Virtues: anti-flatulent, anti-inflammatory, antispasmodic, aromatic, carminative, diaphoretic, rubefacient, stimulant, and checks nausea. Mother Nature made more than three dozen species, and clever gardeners, along with focused botanists, have come up with more hybrids. The Greeks, Romans, and Druids all used mints in sacred rites. Best known as a digestive aid, peppermint's sweet, pleasant taste gives medicinal herbs a good name. Native Americans drank peppermint tea to prevent nausea and fevers. The ubiquitous "after dinner mint" still served widely in restaurants is descended from European royalty regularly drinking this digestive tea after their elongated banquets. Folk uses: heartburn and menstrual pain.

Therapeutic uses: irritable bowel syndrome, depression, motion sickness, sore throat, stimulant, diarrhea, and plays a role in ulcerative colitis and Crohn's disease. Caution: The oil is quite strong and should not be used internally; it may be used as an inhalant or on the temples for headache relief. I've long enjoyed the way the chocolate mint takes over the garden, growing, splaying, and flourishing. (No surprise that mint is associated magically with abundance!)

Psyllium (Plantago ovata) husks, native to Mediterranean region and North Africa. Virtues: alterative, hepatic, laxative, liver and gallbladder support. Effective adjuvant for lowering cholesterol, colon problems, diverticulitis, colitis, constipation, inflammation, irritable bowel syndrome, dysentery, ulcers, and escorting heavy toxic overload from bile out of the body. A main component of psyllium is mucilage, soothing and bulking. As a soluble fiber, intestinal bacteria will react with it, in turn having a healing effect on the stresses and innate strategies of a digestive tract coping with medications, metals from cans, preservatives, and improperly digested foods. Psyllium is an efficient agent to help a compromised intestinal tract decontaminate, nurturing its recovery.

Red Clover (Trifolium pratense) flower, native to Europe and naturalized across the United States, it's also the official Vermont state flower. Virtues: detoxifier, nervine, sedative for nervous exhaustion, pectoral. Possessing a strong concentration of natural estrogens, red clover helps relieve PMS, menopause, and menstrual-related problems. Native Americans expanded the use of red clover for sore eyes and burns; excellent for the skin, especially during childhood diseases. "And for all the hubbub over Hoxsey, it's probably safer than some of the devastating chemotherapies out there." (Duke)

Red Raspberry (Rubus idaeus) leaves and fruit, native to North America and Europe. Virtues: alterative, analgesic, antiemetic, antiseptic, antispasmodic, antiviral, astringent, galactagogue, homeostatic, oxytocic, stimulant, tonic to the female system. Having migrated the world over and readily adopted by indigenous people, red raspberry leaf tea is terrific during pregnancy. According to Hutchens, "…it will strengthen and prevent miscarriage and render parturition less laborious. The infusion will also relieve painful menstruation and aid the flow..." As a homeostatic, it can quell excessive menstruation, is a wonderful tonic for every cycle of womanhood, and is nutritive during all nine months of pregnancy. (Gladstar) After childbirth, it helps decrease uterine swelling. Additionally, red raspberry assists in relief from diarrhea and dysentery for both men and women. Other applications include morning sickness, bowel problems, breast feeding, leucorrhea, hemorrhoids, gastric disorders, prostate problems. (While the berries are less potent, they contain these nutrients too.) Red raspberry leaf tea is delightful to put in a gift basket for a pregnant girlfriend, continuing the mothercraft tradition of sharing teas…

Rosemary (Rosmarinus officinalis) leaf, native to the Mediterranean hills. Virtues: alterative, anodyne, anti-inflammatory, antioxidant, antiseptic, aromatic, astringent, carminative, diaphoretic, nervine, stimulant, stomachic. The ancient Greeks revered rosemary for improving memory and strengthening focus. Mediterranean students wore sprigs to enhance their learning, and European royalty decided the territorial fates of foreign lands while sipping rosemary tea. A rousing, cognitive stimulant, it works on circulation and the pelvic region. Aromatic and tasty, known as a heart tonic, it's good for high blood pressure. An ally to help relieve hysterical depression, diminishes headaches, and assists a student when studying. Other traditional uses also include: gas, edema, gallbladder, gastric disorders, restlessness, hair loss, and prostate problems. Both *Front Pharmacol* and *Biomed Pharmacother*, two scientific journals, reported that for prostate-protecting nutrients, rosemary "...extract has demonstrated anti-prostate cancer activity in preclinical studies." And every cookbook has a number of tasty dishes which feature this hardy little shrub. "There's rosemary, that's for remembrance…" (Shakespeare)

Sage (Salvia officinalis) leaves, native to the Mediterranean. Virtues: alterative, antigalactagogue, antioxidant, antiseptic, antispasmodic, aromatic, astringent, carminative, diaphoretic, digestive, febrifuge, stimulant, vulnerary. Hailed as a culinary delight by European royalty, sage has been used for cooking and as a medicinal staple for over 2,000 years. The tea may be used a gargle, a nerve tonic, and to decrease flatulence. It addresses mental exhaustion, continued focus, and Alzheimer's disease. (Duke) For concentration, combine sage with ginkgo. A seasoning for roasts and soups, and a must for your Thanksgiving turkey.

St. John's Wort (Hypericum perforatum) aerial parts, native to Europe, West Asia, and North Africa. Virtues: alterative, antineoplastic, antispasmodic, astringent, blood purifier, diuretic, nervine, sedative, vulnerary. In Medieval times, St. John's Wort's virtues included being an antidote to evil spirits and demons, which may come from its legendary employment for depression, stress, anxiety, nervous tension, and sleep. Clinical testing confirms it's effective for treating mild to moderate depression. You can add it to various dishes throughout the day and then have an after-dinner cup of tea to address nervous system conditions. It contains hypericin, a compound being researched for use in treating HIV, AIDS, cancer, viruses including herpes, and T-cell counts. Additional applications include arthritis, lung congestion, rheumatism, spasms, and heart problems. As a salve or even solar-infused oil, St. John's Wort has been dabbed on for stretch marks, burns, insect bites, wounds, boils. St. John's Wort has proven to be a quiet, behind-the-scenes friend.

Sarsaparilla (Smilax ornate, Smilax officinalis, Smilax species) root, native to Central America. Virtues: alterative, anti-inflammatory, antiseptic, aromatic, blood purifier, carminative, diaphoretic, diuretic, febrifuge, hepatoprotective, stimulant. Helpful in glandular cleansing, rejuvenation, sexual activity, lethargy, and building up the body's resources. "Extensively employed in secondary syphilis and conditions following the imprudent use of mercury..." (Parke-Davis) This wonderful, spicy root has a taste that continues on when drunk as a tea. In the 1800s, one could visit the local drug store, sit at the counter, and order a sarsaparilla float (ice cream covered in sarsaparilla syrup, sipped through a straw).

Sassafras (Sassafras albidum, sassafras officinale) roots and leaves, native to North America. Virtues: adaptogen, alterative, anodyne, anti-arthritic, anti-inflammatory, diaphoretic, diuretic, stimulant, tonic. The leaves of the sassafras are used in creole cooking known as file powder. Sassafras and sarsaparilla were the two, original, delicious herbs used to make American root beer. A Native American favorite, it was used to dispel a fever. So valuable in activating the body's own healing that when it was carried back to Europe, it was listed in the British Pharmacopoeia. The United States 1865 Dispensatory states, "The complaints for which it has been particularly recommended are chronic rheumatism, cutaneous eruptions, and scorbutic and syphiloid affections." In 1939, Kloss stated, "Useful as a tonic to stomach and bowels. Will relieve gas." In 2007, Kuhn and Winston stated, "Not commonly used, except as a home remedy and beverage tea. The purported toxicity of sassafras as a tea is overstated, and its occasional ingestion in small amounts is not a cause for serious concern. The carcinogen safrole is poorly water-soluble, so very little is consumed in a tea. Avoid the EO [essential oil], capsules, and tincture because of their high safrole content." In 1993, Gladstar stated, "Sassafras, long valued as a 'blood purifier' and 'liver herb,' is an important ingredient of many old-fashioned root-beer drinks. It contains safrole, a very potent plant chemical that is largely insoluble in water (hardly extracted when making tea). When safrole was isolated from the herbs and injected in extremely high doses into laboratory animals, it produced carcinogenic cells. Based on this information, sassafras was banned from use in all soft drinks. (Synthetic chemicals are now used instead.) *It is interesting that the southern United States, where sassafras grows naturally and has been enjoyed as a beverage tea and a blood cleanser for generations, has the lowest rate of cancer in our country.* It is even more interesting to note that there is not one recorded case of sassafras poisoning or of sassafras-related cancer." In 2000, Duke stated, "The aromatic, sweet-tasting sassafras was regarded as a blood-purifying, all-purpose tonic for whatever ails you, including syphilis. The pleasing flavor made it a favored tea on both sides of the Atlantic. For a while, only tobacco topped this eastern North American native as an export to Europe. Sassafras livened up the taste of chewing gum, toothpastes, and beverages (notably root beer) until the 1960s, when research established that one primary chemical in its volatile oil, safrole, causes cancer. The FDA then banned sassafras' use in food unless the safrole is removed." "Sass" was a synthetic drug, a form of Ecstasy, derived from extracts of sassafras. "Sass, a euphoric stimulant also known as Sally, was a new term to some drug abuse experts, who said drug production and slang change constantly. Safrole, derived from sassafras oil, can be used as a precursor to MDMA or Ecstasy, and the U.S. Food and Drug Administration has banned its use in food as a cancer-causing agent." "A suburban woman died after ingesting drug 'sass,' police say." (By Robert McCoppin, *Chicago Tribune*, Nov. 13, 2014) Neither the FDA nor the CDC has listed any deaths from sassafras albidum nor sassafras officinale. Yet this tasty, powerhouse tea is an excellent metaphor for the way the benefits of medicinal herbs have been distorted and maligned. Faithfully handed down in the Western Pharmacopoeia, wise women, like Native Americans, recognized the necessity of reawakening the body's innate wisdom in the spring just as Mother Nature was blooming in the forest. The Native Americans lived so well that the original explorers described them as "remarkable in their physical appearance and good health." The tribal healers knew a springtime tonic was needed, so they used one. Fast forward to late 20th century, the back-to-the-land movement, the renaissance of ancient herbal wisdom, and new age road blocks. A competitor to costly medications and apparatus treatments of inconvenience, one master herbalist from England stated about sassafras, "They've taken away the most effective herbs, so [herbal] practitioners have less to work with." Moreover, enterprising young phytochemists have dabbled and hacked the botanical profiles of medicinal herbs for profit, eager to amplify results from hallucinogenics and rival the black market. Cause-and-effect, building community, valuing nature, and honoring traditions are hardly part of the educational landscape these days, even as we face an advancing algorithm of disease. We do need to learn how to live in a global village, for more reasons than one. It is time to resurrect what tradition has proven right.

Saw Palmetto (Serenoa repens or Serenoa serrulata) berries, native to Southeastern United States. Virtues: adaptogen, alterative, antiseptic, aphrodisiac, sedative, revitalizes male reproductive system, uretic, hormone imbalances, impotency, reproductive organs, infertility, nerve pain, colds, urinary problems. In traditional folk uses, saw palmetto is known as an aphrodisiac and sexual stimulant, and currently ranks as a premium remedy for prostate problems. The two organs of the body that grow for all of one's life are the nose and the prostate. Since most men will probably experience discomfort or a prostate issue because of this continued enlargement, saw palmetto has been verified as a prophylactic to begin taking early in adult life. "Saw palmetto frequently equals and sometimes exceeds pharmaceuticals for treating benign prostate hypertrophy (BPH), the noncancerous enlargement of the prostate that strikes at least half of all men 50 years old and as many as 90 percent of all men 70 years old and up. The condition makes urination difficult, perhaps painful, and leaves a man unable to empty his bladder thoroughly, resulting in frequent visits to the bathroom, especially at night. More than a dozen clinical studies involving almost 3,000 men...[showed] saw palmetto's ability to markedly alleviate BPH symptoms, increasing urinary flow and decreasing the number of sleep-disturbing jaunts to the john—without the libido-reducing side effects of its pharmaceutical rival." (Duke) "Saw Palmetto benefits the prostate by (1) Inhibiting enzymes that convert testosterone into dihydrotestosterone [DHT], a hormone that increases prostate growth, and (2) Supporting healthy cell division and inflammatory response with the prostate. This reduces lower urinary tract symptoms, which include urinary incontinence, needing to urinate too often, or having trouble urinating." (Life Extension) "Valuable in catarrh, chronic bronchitis, acute and chronic laryngitis, asthma and whooping cough...Recently attention has been called to a specially vitalizing action of Saw Palmetto upon the glands of the reproductive apparatus—mammae, ovaries, etc.—hence the value of the drug in atrophy of the uterus and appendages, and of their male analogues, the prostate and testes." (Parke-Davis)

Schizandra Berry (Schisandra chinensis) berries, native to Eastern Asia. Virtues: adaptogen, alterative, antibacterial, astringent, cardioprotective, hepatoprotective, tonic, stimulant. Schizandra is one of the primary *adaptogen* Asian herbs that introduced this Traditional Chinese Medicine virtue to the West. An adaptogen can either invigorate the energy of a body's action or it can calm the energy of a body's action. Just as the body's own wisdom "knows" when to rev up and when to wind down, so too does the adaptogen herb; it assists the body's innate wisdom for healing itself. Schizandra berry stimulates the immune system, revives liver cells after alcohol, drugs, or even hepatitis, avails allergies, and treats depression. Indicated in Chinese medicine for "loss of essence," frequent urination from deficient kidneys issues, deficiency of the spleen, depressed adrenals, stress, and mild digestive disorders. Grind the dried berries into a powder for baking or adding to a smoothie. A great way to get going in the morning is with schizandra berry morning muffins.

Siberian Ginseng/Eleuthero (Eleutherococcus senticosus) roots, native to Eastern Asia. Virtues: adaptogen, anti-depressant (mild), grounding, stimulant, tonic. Eleuthero can be safely used to increase stamina in the face of undue demands and stress, be it physical or mental. It improves memory and adrenal response. It reinforces the immune system while supporting therapy for cancer treatment: increases natural killer and T-helper cells as well as reduces side effects of chemotherapy and radiation. (Kuhn/ Winston) While not as aggressive as panax ginseng, its long-term support (re)builds the body.

Sheep's Sorrel (Rumex acetosa) leaves, native to Europe and Asia. Virtues: anti-inflammatory, aperient, diuretic, litholitic (mild), nutrient, refrigerant, vermicide. With a somewhat lemony flavor in salads, it's necessary in the transformation process of foods, especially with enzymes, helpful with fats. "(The leaves)….may be used advantageously as an article of diet in scurvy." (United States Dispensatory) Within the alternative health community, sheep's sorrel holds a place of honor in the esteemed, anti-cancer, Essiac formula.

Skullcap/Scullcap (Scutellaria lateriflora) aerial parts, native to North America. Virtues: alterative, analgesic, antibacterial, antispasmodic, febrifuge, nervine, sedative. Eclectic physicians adopted skullcap from Native Americans in cases of insomnia, nervous tension, exhaustion, depression, epilepsy, high blood pressure, and spasms. It revivifies the central nervous system after alcohol and drug withdrawal. It's useful when treating seizure disorders, headaches, agitation, hysteria, PMS, urinary problems, and undue sexual desires. The name is reminiscent of the nightcaps worn to bed long ago, a reminder to quiet down.

Slippery Elm Bark (Ulmus fulva) inner bark, native to Eastern North America. Virtues: antacid, antineoplastic, supreme demulcent, emollient, expectorant, strong mucilant, nutritive. In the winter of Valley Forge,

General Washington notified the quartermaster that the soldiers be advised to start eating slippery elm bark. With the deep snow cover that winter, they couldn't dig up root vegetables from the frozen ground, yet this reliable mucilant kept them fed. Whether decocted as a tea or cooked as a porridge, slippery elm is a food that delivers medicinal support. This nutritious demulcent was perfectly suited for the sensitive, inflamed mucous membrane linings of the soldiers' digestive systems, a trying health issue for the Continental Army which was low on food and high on dysentery. Even the Native Americans used the inner bark in a salve against wounds, abscesses, boils, warts, and dermatitis. Internally, benefits gastritis, gastric or duodenal ulcers, colitis, diarrhea, hemorrhoids, constipation, and diverticulitis. It's especially soothing for sore throats, bronchitis, flu, and whooping cough. When added to wild cherry bark, it is a remarkable, wintertime tea. (Note: given the value of the mucilage in slippery elm bark, this one is not for tincturing.)

Spirulina (Spirulina maxima, S. platensis) powdered seaweed algae, S. maxima is native to Central America and S. platensis is native to Africa, Asia, and South America. Virtues: anticancer, alterative, antimicrobial, hepatic, immune-potentiator, stimulant. Known to increase oxygen utilization, this blue-green algae is high in protein and benefits the body in acute cases of colds, flus, and fevers. It's rich in amino acids; GLA (gamma-linolenic acid) is *an omega-6 fatty acid,* found in plant seed oils such as borage oil and evening primrose oil), essential fatty acids, trace minerals, and iron. It even helps curb an appetite. The high amount of chlorophyll soothes detox headaches. For hypoglycemia, using spirulina between meals can stabilize the blood sugar. "Spirulina is a very powerful detoxifying agent. It chelates all types of toxins such as mercury, arsenic, radioactive materials, cadmium, pesticides, and environmental carcinogens, eliminating them from the body." (fulcompany.com) If you and Tom Hanks are castaways on an island, this is the desert-island-pick-superfood you want.

Stevia (Stevia rebaudiana) leaves, native to South America. Virtues: antibacterial, antidiabetic. Tonic and antidepressive can be added to the virtues' list in the sense that if one *stops ingesting the white sugar sold in the marketplace today*, the body is better able to absorb good nutrients and won't have the "sugar-high-sugar-drop-depression" many present-day people get. A green leaf, no-calorie sweetener that is 100 times sweeter than sugar, stevia is safe for a diabetic since the body doesn't recognize it as a carbohydrate. High in chromium, which helps stabilize blood sugar levels, stevia has been shown to help suppress dental caries and can be employed for an obesity protocol. Rather than the powdered white crystals being marketed as "a sugar substitute," try tasting these delightful green leaves when they're brewed as a tea. Pour a tablespoon of the stevia tea into your regular coffee or tea, and experience the difference.

Squawvine (Mitchela repens) berries, leaves, and stalks, native to North America. Virtues: alterative, anti-inflammatory, antiseptic, astringent, diuretic, emmenagogue, galactagogue. Also known as squaw berry and partridge berry, Native American women drank the tea *during their final week of pregnancy* because it was especially helpful "in order to render parturient safe and easy." (Hutchens) Traditionally, squawvine was a uterine tonic since it relieves congestion of the uterus and ovaries, and its antiseptic properties improve a vaginal infection. It can activate the flow of mother's milk, is a deep, natural sedative, and when the time is right, restores menstrual flow. During a workshop, we made a nipple salve combining the squawvine berries, red raspberry leaves, and calendula flowers. **DO NOT USE DURING PREGNANCY.**

Thyme (Thymus vulgaris) leaves, stems, and flowers, native to Europe and Northern Africa. Virtues: alterative, antibacterial, antifungal, antiseptic, antispasmodic, aromatic, carminative, diaphoretic, emmenagogue, expectorant, nervine, parasiticide, rubefacient, vulnerary. Across battlefields and oceans, thyme's been carefully carried in doctor's chests because of its immediate, effective results for chronic respiratory conditions, allergies, and lung congestion. Thyme probably served each invading army well during the heat of battle, when there was no time to adapt to unaccustomed flora and fauna on foreign land. Not only was the tea useful as a general tonic, it also played a role in killing worms, gout, digestion, parasites, gastritis, and bowel problems. It's even helpful in suppressed menstruation. Every cookbook from the 1900s on has a plethora of recipes with thyme. Thyme combines well with garlic, as well as a thyme-parsley-marjoram-chive combo for chicken. Enjoy experimenting with them all. **DO NOT USE DURING PREGNANCY.**

Turkey rhubarb (Rheum palmatum) root, native to Asia. Virtues: astringent, bitter, purgative. It's a cousin to the more common rhubarb, so popular in springtime strawberry-rhubarb pie. Turkey rhubarb encourages smooth peristaltic, muscle movements of the intestines, accelerating stool with the help of beneficial intestinal bacteria. The excretion of waste products can include nitrogenous waste accumulated in patients with renal failure; hence, it has been used to treat patients with kidney issues. Valued for clearing the cause of intestinal irritations, whether diarrhea or dysentery. **DO NOT USE DURING PREGNANCY.**

Turmeric (Curcuma longa) root, native to Southeast Asia. Virtues: Anodyne, antibacterial, anticoagulant, antifungal, anti-inflammatory, antineoplastic, antioxidant, antiviral. Versatile and historic, turmeric has been employed in India as a flavorful culinary spice, a tenacious dye, and a powerful medicinal herb. Known for its use in cleansing, inflammation, arthritis, infections, liver disorders, joint pains, heart issues, and dealing with tumors, in conjunction with warm, stimulating effects on digestion and circulation. It's been proven to help prevent and treat gallstones and as an anti-inflammatory for rheumatoid arthritis. Research has shown that turmeric, with genistein, inhibits the formation of cancer in breast tissue. In further research, the curcumins cut the risk of colon cancers and seem to neutralize cancer-causing compounds; it stops cancerous changes in cells. (Duke) Turmeric assists in regulating blood sugar levels, activating bile flow, and diminishing PMS. Its spicy, bitter flavor makes every curry dish delicious, a classic staple in Ayurvedic cuisine. Turmeric holds an elevated place in both the apothecary's cupboard and on the spice rack.

Valerian (Valerian officinalis) root, native to Europe and Asia. Virtues: alterative, antiseptic, carminative, decongestant, diuretic, galactagogue, nervine, sedative. Employed as a nerve tonic, valerian has traditionally been applied to "hysterics," PTSD, healing an ulcerated stomach, insomnia, and even in small doses, soothing a baby with colic. It can curb the number of times someone awakens in the middle of the night. In 1653, Culpepper said, "The root of Valerian boiled with liquorice, raisins, and aniseed, is singularly good for those that are short-winded, and for those that are troubled with the cough, and helps to open the passages, and to expectorate phlegm easily…It is of a special virtue against the plague, the decoction thereof being drank, and root being used to smell to…" And cats like it almost as much as catnip!

Watermelon (Citrullus lanatus) seeds, native to Africa. Virtues: antioxidants, nutrients, and the seeds are an outstanding diuretic. They've been used for dropsy and gout. They can soothe inflammation and increase circulation to the kidneys when addressing a congested system. "Chiefly diuretic and demulcent, but is likewise a mild hepatic and intestinal stimulant. Useful in irritation of kidneys or bladder, especially in retention of urine due to cold." (Parke-Davis) The seeds don't have to be spit out; you can just munch, crunch, and eat them.

White Willow Bark (Salix alba) bark, native to Europe, Central Asia, and Northern Africa. Virtues: analgesic, anodyne, anthelmintic, anti-inflammatory, anti-periodic, antispasmodic, diaphoretic, febrifuge. Even the ancient Greek physician Dioscorides employed white willow bark for pain and inflammation, and its virtues have been counted, assayed, examined, and dissected for thousands of years. While both meadowsweet and white willow bark were tested for pain relief because of their salicin, it was Bayer who unveiled its new product extracted from white willow bark in the 19th century, coining the name "aspirin." Associated with heartburn, occasional fevers, ague, arthritis, colds, gout, fever, earaches, and ovarian pain, the body metabolizes salicin into salicylic acid, which cools inflammation and reduces pain. Versatile and easy, a cup of white willow bark tea can accompany almost any illness.

Wild Cherry Bark (Prunus virginiana) bark, native to North America and Central America Virtues: Alterative, antiasthmatic, anticatarrhal, antispasmodic, antitussive, astringent, bitter, carminative, expectorant, nervine, parasiticide, gentle sedative, stomachic. Luden's still sells "Wild Cherry" cough drops because the tea proved to be a useful expectorant, colonial Americans decocted it for cough elixirs, and early pastilles were made of licorice and wild cherry bark. Wild cherry bark benefits bronchial disorders caused by the hardened accumulation of mucus. Folk uses include heart palpitations, tuberculosis, dyspepsia, fevers, and diarrhea. Many people from warmer climates, like the Caribbean and South America, have relocated to the Northeast. These newcomers need adjustment to the four seasons, as those first few winters can ravage and debilitate bodies acclimated to year-round sunshine. A good protocol of prevention would be drinking wild cherry bark tea about twice a week, beginning in October and continuing through March. If a cold ensues, drink more tea as needed. It's flavorful and combines well with slippery elm bark for a scratchy-throat kind of cough.

Wild Yam (Dioscorea villosa) root, native to North America [Other species are native to China]. Virtues: Anti-inflammatory, antispasmodic, blood purifier, cholagogue, diaphoretic. The wise woman tradition used wild yam for regulating hormone production, and researchers praised its value in the development of synthetic hormones, a scientific advance necessary in the creation of birth control pills. "…At one time this herb was the sole source of the chemicals that were used as the raw materials for contraceptive hormone manufacture." (Hoffman) It is associated with glandular balance, menstrual distress, menopause, and endometriosis. Additionally, arthritis, bowel spasms, nausea, pain, rheumatism, inflammation, nervousness, and ulcers have been aided with wild yam.

Wormwood (Artemisia absinthium) leaves and/or flowering tops, native to Eurasia. Virtues: Alterative, anthelmintic, anti-inflammatory, bitter tonic, carminative, febrifuge, stomachic. Traditional uses of wormwood included counteracting poisoning from toadstools and hemlock, allaying food poisoning, dispelling intestinal worms, aiding and purifying the digestive tract, treating liver and gallbladder ailments, and stimulating the appetite. Dr. Duke says, "Distillers made it the primary constituent of absinthe, an addictive, narcotic nineteenth-century liqueur notorious for damaging both the brain and the nerves [so] that it was eventually banned (well, almost)…Straight thujone, another of the phytochemicals, supposedly is a hallucinogenic brain depressant that inhibits the ability to breathe." David Hoffman says, "Wormwood has been used in a wide range of conditions, most of which have been vindicated by analysis of the herbs. The apparent 'cure-all' nature of this herb can largely be explained in the fundamental impact that its bitter action has on the body…It is primarily used as a bitter and therefore has the effect of stimulating and envigorating the whole of the digestive process. It is often used where there is indigestion…"

Yarrow (Achillea millefolium) flowers, native to Europe Virtues: Alterative, antiseptic, astringent, blood purifier, diaphoretic, diuretic, homeostatic, vulnerary. Named for none other than the mythic, military hero Achilles, ancient Greek soldiers regularly carried yarrow into battle as a warrior's talisman. Influenced by its legendary wound-healing properties, soldiers secured these hardy flowers for battlefield lacerations, dysentery, and emotional support. Yarrow deals with fevers, lowers blood pressure, stimulates digestion, counters inflammation and tissue swelling, remedies hemorrhage, stays bleeding from lungs, and post-childbirth, promotes feminine healing. **DO NOT USE DURING PREGNANCY.**

Yellowdock (Rumex crispus) roots, native to Europe and Asia. Virtues: alterative, aperient, cholagogue, mildly purgative. Originally from the Old World, yellowdock became a favorite with Native Americans for eruptive skin diseases and ailments of the eyes, ears, nose, and throat. An astringent and blood purifier useful in treating diseases of the lymphatic system, scrofula, glandular tumors, swelling, and speeds up elimination of metals from the body. Updating for modern usage, if you have eaten many canned foods, yellowdock is good for eliminating the trace metals. "...appears to be of service in strumous diathesis." (Parke-Davis) Yellowdock nourishes the spleen, liver, and bile flow.

When on a walkabout, I've found in the City: thyme, poke, sassafras, dandelion, yellowdock, burdock, plantain, chickweed, Joe Pye weed, bugleweed, echinacea, bella donna, mullein, mints, ginkgo, white pine, purslane, wood sorrel, red clover, and sunflowers, to name a few.

The Boston Tea Party and Functional Liberty Teas

In the 1600s and 1700s, coveted teas and spices traveled halfway around the world, hand-picked, laboriously curated, carefully dried, packed individually, and delicately loaded onto English East India ships, bound for the New World. Still learning what to forage in New England forests, the colonial mothers relied on these shipments from Great Britain for their medicinal and culinary herbs.

I admire the Pilgrims who braved the New World, following their beliefs, on their own path. Squaring off against the world's strongest military force at that time, those underprepared American forefathers and foremothers stood up to the excessive British taxation and suppressive laws. In one of history's greatest pieces of political theatre, patriots dressed up in Indian leather britches, painted their faces, put feathers in their hair, and raided a merchant ship in Boston Harbor, tossing 342 chests of tea overboard on December 16, 1773. Quite perturbed that this "bunch of rabble" insulted the crown by assaulting such precious cargo, the colonies were told, "No more shipments of spices and teas." (Remember, the colonial goodwives could not just shop in a different supermarket nor place another order on Amazon.) But Yankee know-how prevailed, and the courageous pluck of the marauding Boston Tea Party patriots extended to their patriot wives. Determined to carry on a proper home, the goodwives readily began procuring what was growing in the New World. The colonial mothers declared their own liberty by making "Liberty Teas," using the herbs found in the New England forests. It was a sign of independence to serve a "Liberty Tea" to one's guests, and to cook and caretake with New World botanicals. With bull-dog confidence and the arrogance of a youthful nation, the colonies declared their independence from England on July 4, 1776. In turn, General Washington ordered the writing of a New England materia medica for the continental army's apothecaries, and veneration for women's work in the New World was born.

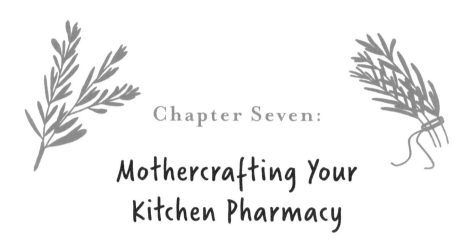

Chapter Seven

Mothercrafting Your Kitchen Pharmacy

Trending diets: Paleolithic, Keto, Mediterranean, South Beach diet, hyper-drive-metabolic diet, intermittent fasting diet, toughest-workout diet, and a few "no-changes-to-anything-and-lose-40-pounds-in-a-month" diets. They are about weight loss, directed at a population with ready access to fast foods and gourmet celebrities. *"How come the Standard-American-Diet (SAD) produces so many overweight people?"* An open-ended question for a psychology class, with loopholes and secondary characters.

More people are becoming diabetic, allergic to gluten, developing auto-immune illnesses, acknowledging autism, obesity, and it's assumed now, that if you're over 65, you're on two to six medications daily. Yet our ancestors lived without preservatives and chemical medications; what happened? Better to do a comparison-contrast of what we were born with and where we are now.

After the Garden of Eden, hunters and gatherers nested in caves. Annemarie Colbin did tremendous work about what they did for food and the history of traditional diets: In North America, meal times included moose, caribou, buffalo, fish, other animals, berries, bark, mosses, and plant roots. There were fruits and nuts, and a few cultivated plants such as corn, beans, squash, amaranth, sunflower seeds, pumpkins, and zucchini. Additionally, in more arid places, mice, rats, reptiles, and even insects were eaten. In South America, many kinds of birds, fish, dried fish eggs, and sea kelp—a highly nutritious food source—were standard tribal fare. Vegetables included potatoes, sweet potatoes, squash, corn, beans, quinoa, tomatoes, peppers, and peanuts. Fruits included coconuts, figs, pomegranates, peaches, grapes, and strawberries.

People were eating plants as soon as they distinguished the edible ones. Through patient trial and error, humans winnowed out plant kingdoms, categorized them by medicinal virtues, played with culinary spices, and respectfully left the rest to other, foraging species. I suspect humankind had a keener sense of smell in the stone age. Anyone who's owned a dog or cat will notice how they always sniff at a new plate of food. From the first whiff, an animal knows whether it's edible or not. And they're right. Likewise, before pollutants and preservatives corrupted our palates, humans probably walked the forest, plucked a new leaf, sniffed and nibbled, and knew instantaneously whether they'd procured food. (We've retained the scents for burnt and spoiled foods.) Moreover, our palates delighted in the flavor of bitters. The bitters category of herbs gets our gastric juices flowing. (That sprig of parsley on your plate at dinner awakens your digestive system.) In the past, the envelope on our tongues hadn't been pushed with vessels of sugar and white flour, sweet cakes in lieu of garden greens, and slabs of highly salted animal meat. In cave days, an apple provided the same burst of sweet sensation that today's society gets from a monstrous slice of chocolate cake. For our earliest ancestors, plucking small leaves and digging stately roots were the norm, adding up to savory moments throughout the day. While global cultures have evolved in the last ten-thousand years, our bodies have remained nearly the same, still designed for our humble, Paleolithic start in this world. Yet our food sources, daily routines, contact with nature, and spiritual discourse metamorphized into a techno-social-media-metropolitan routine, with nary a milepost to guide us. Traditionally, after waking up, men picked up their bows and arrows for hunting. After tying their papooses on their backs, women picked up gathering baskets for wildcrafting. Days were spent walking, standing, bending, carrying, running, listening, analyzing, and evaluating nature, her plants, her animals, and her landscape. And they had to be really good at what they did; it was called survival. Darwin did us a favor by cataloguing these early efforts and publishing a major law of earth's evolution: survival of the fittest. Early tribal clans learned about learning, with comparison, contrast, application, analysis, and evaluation. In the 21st century, our bodies still wake up with this embedded blueprint. Today, many a hunter wakes up to his caffeine addiction, may eat a sugary donut, walks to a car, rides 45 minutes to work through choked traffic or rides 45 minutes on a subway train scouting the landscape for muggers. He arrives at an office, sits at a desk for eight hours staring into computer blue light, leaves work, walks to the pub for alcoholic co-regulation, gets back in a car or subway for another tense ride home, still alert because the muggers know people are more off guard by the day's end. At home, he sits in front of a television or computer for another few hours. So many of his instincts and urges have been suppressed all day. A gatherer's day may be the about same, while female hormones rage and flair up against the chemicals, pollutants, and interfering city lights. She must carry a pregnancy to term through this constrained, high tech, de-natured habitat.

In cosmological readings, it is suggested that illness is a way for us to reconnect with our own bodies; it's an excuse to go inward and rethink one's self again, and again, and again…

Those many moons ago, very happy my body was finally healing, there were still prefixes and suffixes to be amended to my new routine, and that was when I discovered engineering schedules.

"Let food be thy medicine and medicine be thy food."

— Hippocrates

My body had changed. I went to see another doctor who talked me into a complete physical in order to ascertain my correct diet. Still a poor college student (working one or two jobs per semester to pay my living expenses), the $150 price tag for this in the 1970s was more than I paid each month for rent. (No health insurance in those days.) But I needed more information, so I thought it was worth it. The doctor listened to my heart, listened when I inhaled deeply, questioned my bowel movements, and charted my restored menses. He stuck little electrodes across my torso, took some "readings," and came up with a diet plan for me. At the time, I shared a house far out in Queens with four college roommates. I got up at 6:00 a.m. to ride the subway for over an hour on weekdays to get to my law clerk's job in Brooklyn Supreme Court. After working all morning, I would ride the uptown subway midday for almost an hour to get to my afternoon and evening classes at Fordham. Then, for the third time in a day, I'd ride the subway for another hour to get back to Queens after 10:00 p.m. and do homework. All that subway time was spent studying for school; every minute was stacked up against my future commitments. When the doctor presented me with his prescriptive meal plan to resolve my discomforts, his diet listed three meals I was supposed *to cook daily.*

Putting aside that I shared a kitchen with roommates, how was I supposed to get up earlier and start cooking? By what method was I supposed to inflame, stew, and simmer a meal, midday, riding the subway from Brooklyn to Manhattan? Where would I find a stove at 5:00 p.m. on my college campus for his requisite dinner? On this list, the only "meal" that I could prepare and take with me was "15 raisins and 4 tablespoons of cream cheese." I stared at this regimen and said, "I can't do this." Cutting me off, he told me to "just make it work." I was a young girl, navigating my way into adulthood, didn't know about setting boundaries, but I sure felt mine had just been violated. I swallowed, paid my bill, made a couple of those meals on the weekends, and later vowed that if I ever gave advice, it would fit into a *real* person's life.

> "Over 70% of the world's population today still rely on herbs for their medicine."
>
> — The World Health Organization

By developing your own herbal protocols, you take charge of your health and turn all of your meals into "functional foods." You can drink herbal teas, cook with herbal leaves, roots, twigs, bark, berries, flowers, and seeds to your foods, and infuse medicinal oils, and use tinctures and glycerites. Heating, stewing, grilling, fricasseeing, and tossing salads with outstanding medicinal value are simply part of making a recipe. The basics of herbalism are akin to cooking: you and your kitchen witch can begin in your kitchen, reviving the cooking magic of ancient herbalism.

Today, mom-and-pop health food stores are loaded with recycled hippies, all waiting to answer your questions and help you get started.

Plants Versus Industrialized Nutrients: The Roadway without Excipients

Rooting out Mother Nature's original intention for her Garden of Eden means using the body's innate wisdom of storing, recycling, shifting, and layering nutrients; you're employing the body's own sequencing. There is neither one food source nor plant that has all the nutrients needed in a day. Nature expects us to search the forest daily, finding something here and something else there, each food fueling our bodies' needs. In 1937, Hungarian Albert Szent-Gyorgyi received the Noble Prize in Physiology for isolating vitamin C, the first vitamin, and for discovering the components of cellular digestion. The biological combustion process includes chaperone proteins attached to all nutrients, which escort the nutrients into the right receptor sites located throughout the body. Without this chaperone protein from plants, an isolated (inorganic) nutrient may just be swallowed by the body and then excreted by the body.

The mothercrafting of meals means using healthy botanicals daily to create your own functional foods. Recipes of old favorite dishes, into which you mix these whole plants, make marvelous delivery systems to begin with. Amplify your mealtimes with medicinal herbs; this is evolutionary herbalism.

Beginning with capsules, tinctures, and teabags from the health food store is just fine. Capsules and tinctures are portable; they go anywhere. Healing in nature's time, you can control and vary your dosages. Ask the store owner to recommend good brands. You can also choose from a number of reliable herbal tea brands whose formulations have been confirmed. Some tea bags have only one herb in the bag; you can cut open the tea bag and use the twigs and leaves from there, or just leave them inside the bag. If the store sells the herbs in bulk, all the better. Plan to try them in several different ways, bulk, capsule, tincture. You can initiate your practice on your kitchen table, with what you buy from your health food store or plucked from a reputable, online site. When listening to your body, one delivery system will work better than another, different combinations of plants and systems will be effective, specific times during the day will improve the outcome, and a gradual increase in healthiness will prevail.

To Begin

- For **capsules,** begin with one after breakfast and one after lunch per day. Take as capsules or insert them into foods. (You can even open a capsule and sprinkle ¼ or ½ into some yogurt or applesauce just to experiment with. This can also be done for a child.) You can either buy capsules from the store or make your own formulations to address your health issues. After a week, increase to two capsules after breakfast and lunch as needed.

- For tinctures, begin with 10 to 20 drops after breakfast and 10 to 20 drops after lunch. Take as drops or insert them into foods. You can also begin with 2 to 8 drops in some yogurt or applesauce for a child. After a week, increase to 20-30 drops after breakfast and lunch as needed.

- For **tea bags,** begin with one cup in the morning, and one cup midday. Drink them as teas or insert the tea contents into foods. (Increase cups per day as needed.)

- After you understand plant medicine and your own body's responses, you can make your own capsules, tinctures, or teas with your own combinations (formulations). Again, initially try them using the quantities listed above before you increase your dosages.

- **You can mix these dosages into the foods you are already eating.** Consider also that you may have one health issue for which you prefer taking capsules and tinctures, another health issue for which you like mixing your powdered herbs (open a capsule and mix it into food), and sometimes it's good to drink cups of tea (pour them into any soup or batter). These judgement calls are based on your tastes, frequency of necessity, and the kinds of the foods you are eating. (Mothercraft 101)

The health food industry is always scampering around to find *new* delivery systems for their herbal extracts, synthetic constituents, nutritional facsimiles, and techno-brews. Given that you can neither patent nor copyright a weed growing on the side of the road (think: dandelion), what works for large-scale corporations is devising formulas, with parts both natural *and* inorganic. To register a product, corporations need only add something outside the botanical floral compound (think 10 milligrams of vitamin C), and suddenly, *it's a formula.* A formula can be measured, registered, and argued about in court. So, in order to protect their sizable investments, big brands in the health food industry wouldn't invest in a single herb by which to gauge their bottom line. They've come up with a clever Plan B: protein bars, gummies, powders, phosphorescent tablets, health chips, multi-formula capsules, combo tinctures, and spray-ons. Undoubtedly some of these are effective for health purposes. Yet long-term, they're more expensive and may not deliver as much as the complete, nutritional matrix of the plant. When working with whole herbs, your body's recovery is likely to come sooner. When working with the delivery systems you are accustomed to (your morning, afternoon, and evening meals), it's more likely for you to sustain your new, long-term regimen.

Sales and Marketing: Brand Name Extracts

The idea of making an extract is that a significant chemical from a plant should be singled out, extracted, and then potentiated. A good example of this is the curcumin extracted from the herb turmeric. Standardized extracts are touted as "better" because they have only the "good" ingredient from that plant designated to fix a health issue. However, Mother Nature adds in cofactors for her own reasons. She has included in her plants chemicals that act as digestive aids, chaperone proteins, nutrients to balance overreactions, and sometimes, blockers to absorption for other botanical ingredients because the body signals when it's fed up and doesn't need any more of an appointed chemical. But the manufacturers remove these cofactors in order to patent their own products.

(The term *extract* is used in another way in herbalism: it describes an herb that will be tinctured; the medicinal constituents will be extracted from the plant usually by the menstruum of alcohol. This is a more potent liquid dosage than a simple cup of tea. Technically, you can also say that medicinal constituents are extracted from a plant by the menstruum of water when making a cup of tea.)

Mothercrafting Apothecary's Guide: How To Prepare Herbs (Delivery Systems)

Making Tea.

1. **Infusion** (steeping). **Leaves and flowers** can be steeped in a teacup. *Place a heaping teaspoon* (that's where the measurement originated from!) into a strainer, in a teacup, *pour boiling hot water* over the tea leaves or flowers, cover (a small saucer will do), and *let steep for 10 to 25 minutes*. Remove the tea strainer from the cup and sip or add to a recipe.

2. **Decoction** (slow-boil). **Roots, bark, twigs, seeds, and berries** can be slow-boiled in a pot on the stove. Bring 2 to 3 cups of water to a boil. As the water begins to boil, turn the flame down to its *lowest, slow simmer*. Place *a heaping teaspoon* of the tea into the pot. Cover the pot and *let slow simmer for 10 to 15 minutes. Turn off the flame* completely and let the mixture *steep for another 10 to 30 minutes*. Pour the freshly made tea through a strainer into a teacup or add to a recipe.

For either an infusion or a decoction, you can multiply the cups of water and the teaspoons of herbs. For example, suppose you enjoy a nice, big cup of skullcap or hops right before bed. Make a pot of 7 to 8 cups of the tea, and drink it as needed over the next several nights. Or, if it is wintertime, and you're working on immune system building, make 7 to 8 cups of echinacea and use it as needed during the week in various recipes. The body likes "a sip here, and a sip there."

3. **Electuary.** A medicinal herb mixed with honey or fruit pulp. (This works particularly well for making a cough syrup.) Example: Honey with turmeric. For a one-pound jar of honey, mix in one heaping Tablespoon of powdered turmeric. Let it sit in a dark closet for at least a week. Each day, shake the jar for about 60 seconds for the honey to draw out the medicinal

constituents. By the week's end, begin spooning this honey-turmeric electuary over cereals and oatmeal, or just have a teaspoon of it. You can even bake with it. (Hint: Add a pinch of ginger to the honey and turmeric, for flavor and enhancing the potency of the turmeric's benefits.)

4. **Herbal oils.** Choose a good food-grade oil—olive, avocado, sesame, soybean, sunflower, peanut, almond, or walnut—to add your herbs to. An infused oil is one more way to add antidotes and remedies to your diet. (Infused oils can also be used for making beauty products.)

Good choices for food-grade oil infusions include basil, bay, chives, cilantro, dill, marjoram/oregano, rosemary, tarragon, thyme, and basil. (Thyme, oregano, and basil make a nice, traditional, Italian cooking combination.) Other things, like citrus peel, add even more flavor.

Making the oil.

- Gather the herbs, glass bottles or jars, chopping knives, large spoon, sauce pan, and strainer or cheese cloth.

- If using freshly gathered herbs, rinse off and let them dry for a few hours before using. (Water left on herbs interferes with distillation.)

- Sterilize clean glass bottles or jars by boiling them in water for 5-10 minutes. Allow containers to air-dry.

- Chop the herbs into smaller pieces. Add them to bottles. Fresh herbs take up more space in the bottles than dried herbs. Roots and bark are more potent; therefore you need less than flowers or leaves.

- Fill your container approximately 1/4 of the way with herbs. Heat oil over low heat in a saucepan for 2 to 4 minutes. Pour oil into the bottle/jar over the herbs. Leave the herbs in the bottle/

jar for another 24 hours. (You may need to wipe the cap, as water from fresh herbs will condense there.)

- If using fresh herbs, strain them out of oil by pouring the oil from container through a strainer or cheesecloth into another bottle. Dried herbs can remain in oil, but oil will stay fresher for longer if they are strained out. (Sometimes it's attractive to see a few stems and flowers floating around.)

- Once herbs are removed, allow the oil to stay in a cool, dark spot for 2 to 3 days before using.

5. **Making Tinctures.** Take fresh or dried herbs, place in a sterile, glass jar with a lid (preferably a dark glass, amber or blue), and cover the mixture with 1 part water (a good ratio to use to ensure water-soluble constituents are extracted) to 4 parts alcohol of vodka, brandy, or gin (about two inches higher than the herbs). A vegetable glycerin, while not as potent, may be used in lieu of alcohol (the ratio for glycerin is two parts glycerin to three parts water). The sweetness in glycerin is appealing for a child's tincture, as well as for people who prefer no alcohol. You can find vegetable glycerin in a health food store.

- Fresh herbs have more life force, and the advantage of tincturing is to preserve that freshness. Dried herbs can be easier to handle, and you may not be able to find all the fresh herbs you want nearby. Finely chop the plants before placing them in the menstruum. Put the jar on a dark shelf for 3-4 weeks. Label and date your mixture. Shake the mixture twice daily for a minute to help draw out the medicinal constituents.

- After 3-4 weeks, strain the mixture through cheesecloth into another glass jar. (Wring out all the liquid you can from the cheesecloth.) Pour the liquid into a tincture bottle, and use 10 to 40 drops 1-4 times daily.

- Tinctures are renown for "lasting so much longer" than the dried plants. A word of caution here. You really don't want a tincture that has sat in your cupboard for three years; you're not getting the value of it if you only use a few drops once in a while. Use each one up in about six to eight months.

There is this supposition out there that in order to be an herbalist, you are "required" to make tinctures. That is not the case. There are a number of good tincture brands in the marketplace already, and it will save you time if you simply buy one or two, especially when you are getting started with holistic health. Making your own tinctures is less expensive than buying them, so if you plan to use one long term, than it is practical to make a batch for yourself. Granted, tinctures are portable and good when travelling; sometimes you cannot brew a tea nor cook. Another part of the equation is that if you already using two or three herbs daily mixed into your recipes, or even grinding up herbs and making your own capsules, you may want to include a few tinctures in your regimen. They are easily added into foods or drinks by the dropper-full. These choices are all worth considering when creating your protocol.

6. **Poultice.** A hot, soft, moistened, solid portion of mashed herbs (sometimes with flour) is made into a paste and spread on a muslin or white cloth (a man's handkerchief works nicely) and applied for ½ hour to two hours on a sore or inflamed area of the body to relieve pain and inflammation. A poultice can also be used to draw out toxins, blood poisoning, venomous bites, help heal a wound, or send comfort to a particular internal organ (intestines, liver, or womb). The cloth can be presoaked in very warm water so when it's applied to the body, the capillaries become dilated, and the blood flow is increased. A second cotton layer can cover the poultice to reduce heat loss. (Either plantain, comfrey, or yarrow always work well for anything related to skin abrasion.)

7. Which Powdered Herbs or Teas to Add to Your Recipes?

Narrow down the health issue you want to begin with and read about it. Even if you have compounded health issues or comorbidities or debilitating chronic systemic questions, pick one health problem to inaugurate your regimen. What was the first health issue that bothered you? Period cramps? Springtime hay fever? Fall hay fever? Rheumatoid arthritis? Constant gas? Low energy? Think about your health issue, what you initially took for it, and how your body reacted. Did another symptom appear, or get worse? Did you start taking something for that side effect, and then something else was added, and one more thing added, and ten years later, you have various aches, pains, and conditions to be juggled, confronted, and minimized every day? Or perhaps there's one issue that is "the loudest"; look at that health issue. Your issue could be as simple as wanting to cut down from five cups of coffee a day to one cup of decaf. Cutting down on caffeine is a health issue, as are cutting down on sugar, wanting to sleep through the night, not breaking out in acne during a menstrual cycle, not getting triggered into stress when other people unload on you, and sometimes feeling "possessed" unless you satisfy a sweet tooth. Decide which recipes are the easiest to begin adding medicinal vegetables to. You'll find this experimenting, discovering, and seasoning is also *adventuring*.

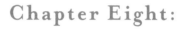

Chapter Eight:

Mothercrafting Your Own Recipes/ Healing Delivery Systems

Today's kitchens usually contain:

- canned soups
- canned tuna fish
- jars of tomato sauce
- bags of white sugar
- bags of white flour
- frozen peas
- frozen spinach
- frozen potatoes
- frozen ice pops
- vanilla, chocolate, and other, razzle-dazzle, whoopee ice creams
- four kinds of soda
- milk (cow's)
- cheeses - cheddar, muenster, gouda
- cream (dairy)
- eggs

- crackers—three kinds, all salty
- loaf of white bread
- loaf of rye
- ground hamburger meat
- beef, three cuts
- chicken
- mayo
- mustard
- barbecue sauce
- hot sauce
- serious cayenne
- big jar of peanut butter
- grape jelly
- cake baking mixes
- cookie baking mixes
- waffle baking mixes
- banana bread baking mixes
- cornbread baking mixes
- biscuit baking mixes
- zucchini baking mixes
- peanut butter baking mixes
- chocolate chip cookie baking mixes
- fudge baking mixes
- triple-sugared breakfast cereals in super-king-sized boxes
- grains-oats, rice, rye, buckwheat, cornmeal
- coffee
- expresso
- black tea bags
- orange-aid juice boxes
- fruit punch juice boxes
- strawberry-kiwi juice boxes

- high vitamin-C juice boxes
- apples, in season
- blueberries, in season
- strawberries, in season
- bananas
- occasional broccoli
- occasional cauliflower
- frozen dinners of every genus, type, class, and brand: meat, chicken, fish, pizza, lasagna, pastas, chili, and plenty of side dishes

Store-bought canned soups: The directions usually tell you to pour the can of soup into a pot. Then, fill the can with water, and add it to the soup contents already in the pot. Instead of filling the soup can with just water, add in *a can of herbal tea*, whichever tea will address the health issue you're working on. Historically, all the botanicals now identified as medicinal herbs were originally pulled from the forest to go into the collective pot for everyone in the tribe to eat. They were eating their "treatments" every day. Making vegetable soup, is really easy; it's already ready for medical vegetables! For example, if it's winter, fill that second soup can with echinacea or Oregon grape root tea. Each is an immune system booster and fits in with a vegetable soup flavor. Just like other recipes, you figure out what-goes-with-what. Slippery elm would be great to add to a butternut squash soup to ease a sore throat or irritated intestinal tract. A sea food soup can take rosemary or thyme, and chicken soup a great base for burdock, yellowdock, or wild yam.

> Starting simple: For healthier eating, incorporate the medicinal herbs right into the foods in your present diet. Over time, you'll have adjusted your diet and lifestyle.

If you need to, you can adjust the seasoning, yet skip the salt, sugar, or anything on the off-limits list.

Canned tuna fish: sprinkle in 1/8 tsp of a powdered herb or 6 drops of a tincture appropriate to taste for fish.

Jars of tomato sauce: They usually have added sugar, so you could begin by adding ¼ powdered tsp of gymnema to block the taste of sugar as well as help control blood sugar for both the type 1 and type 2 diabetic. Another teaspoon of a (powdered) leaf, flower, root, or bark can be mixed in. Or, add in an herbal tea; just remember, it will thin out the sauce.

Bags of white sugar: whatever the recipe calls for, only add ½ the amount. As the body detoxifies and begins absorbing more minerals, there is less of a sweet tooth. You can add a tad more spices to your recipe to enhance flavoring. (Begin trying honey or stevia in your recipes.)

Bags of white flour: It's best to begin transitioning to other kinds of flour: whole wheat, almond, rice, corn, quinoa, or sorghum. As you transition, make the recipe with ½ white flour and ½ a healthier flour.

Frozen peas, spinach, potatoes, or other vegetable dishes: These are perfect for adding in a culinary herb for taste as well as health: tarragon, kelp, cinnamon, sage, or bay are just a few. You can also add an herb that's not usually culinary, but has medicinal value for you, for example, an herb for the female system. Red raspberry leaves can be added to vegetable dishes as well as wild yam root. Or just sprinkle in ½ tsp of the powder or mix in ten drops of the tincture to these frozen veggies.

Ice creams: Take advantage of our how the alternative health food industry has grown. People still like fun foods. There're many dairy-free, new ice creams flavors out there—try them all! A personal favorite is a big dish of coconut-milk vanilla ice cream with freshly picked chocolate mint leaves atop. Divinely delicious.

Sodas: For a sweet drink, try real juice. (Also, try ¼ glass of juice to ¾ glass of water.) Do not be fooled by "diet" sodas; those artificial sweeteners come with cauldrons of serious side effects and disorders. Briefly, drinking soda contributes to liver disease, heart disease, high blood pressure, stroke, diabetes, and has been linked to kidney disease. (https://universityhealth-news.com/daily/nutrition/what-does-soda-do-to-your-body/)

Cow's milk: No animal on earth continues drinking milk after it has been weaned from its mother, *except for humans*. Most humans stop producing the enzyme lactase, necessary to digest dairy, around the age of four. In Mother Nature's book, when a human baby has been weaned from its mother, it doesn't need that milk-digesting enzyme, lactase, anymore because it's time to eat growing up, solid foods. The following are a list of complaints that have been linked to dairy: hives, sinusitis, allergies, heart disorders, impaired digestion, diarrhea, acne, gas and bloating, body odor, constipation, hyperactivity, colitis, headaches, fatigue, anger, depression, congestion, irritability, excess mucus, and malabsorption. Moreover, the antibiotics, pesticides, growth hormones (Bovine somatotropin (bST) and other commercial chemicals the cow ingested do wind up in the cow's milk. "When these people (after early childhood) consume milk, the lactose in it *does* simply stay in their intestines. It is eventually digested not by them, but by the bacteria that live in the human digestive tract (which causes bloating and gas)." (Krogh). What has been noted is that the original populations who react the most to dairy products are from Africa, Asia, and lastly, Eastern Europe. The traditional diets of these populations do not include dairy. But we do know that Northern Europe is where humans began including milk in their diets, and it appears that over time, the human bodies of those descendants may be trying "to adapt." Note that after 10,000 years, the body has hardly changed.

There are many, tasty, non-dairy substitutes on our supermarket shelves these days: almond milk, cashew milk, coconut milk, soy milk, oat milk, and rice milk. They each add a distinctive flavor to a recipe. It's delightful to taste a previous recipe with an updated flavor.

Cheeses and cream: Start trying the many, new varieties of non-dairy cheeses and cream. While these non-dairy cheeses and cream don't have the exact same texture which affects cooking, play with them until you know how they'll perform in each recipe.

Eggs: Nearly as versatile as a cosmic herbal smoothie, feel free to experiment with your scrambled eggs and omelets. One of the great things about eating eggs is they're always made fresh, right before they're served. Just as spinach and mushrooms can be stirred into any egg dish, add in about a tsp of chopped leaves or flowers to what you are making. 10 drops from a tincture also do well.

Crackers: Begin by adding a topping that includes a few drops of a tincture or small amount of a powdered medicament mixed in. I know a father who mixes herbs for focusing with peanut butter and gives it to his son on a favorite cracker every morning. The teacher even remarked how much better the son was doing! Use almond butter, cashew butter, non-dairy cream cheese, and even a bean-pesto spread for adding some antidote plants to.

Loaves of white bread and rye: A sandwich is a clever, culinary creation. Versatile and tasty, one-stop-eating. Adding in a few tincture drops on the bread or even a ¼ tsp of a green herb to a chicken salad spread can continue your health regimen midday. If making toast, non-dairy butter and your local honey are a great combo. By ingesting the friendly local honey made by the friendly local bees, you are acclimating your body to the friendly local pollen. Especially when moving to a new location, it's always best to immerse one's self in the local produce and honey. This will cut down on the body's allergic responses.

Ground hamburger meat: *What an opportunity for formulation.* Meat loaf is usually hamburger meat mixed any of the following: parsley, black pepper, chopped onions, tarragon, basil, chives, vegetable stock, and bread crumbs. That seasoning is enough to carry a variety of healing herbs in the mixture, and the "crunchy" texture of meatloaf lends itself to some cut roots and seeds. Add 1-2 tsp of an appropriate root or bark to chopped mushrooms and onions.

Beef, three cuts: When seasoning, add in powdered herbs. If making a stew, let the beef slow boil in a pot of an herbal tea. This "stew tea" can be brewed at different strengths. Many people eat a large portion of meat for dinner, so remember, it's not the time to add energy herbs. A few drops of a tincture can be added into a steak sauce.

Chicken: Good old chicken soup. Take a huge pasta-pot, pour in seven-nine cups of water, use a favored herb for colds and flu, make the tea, and when the tea is done, add in chicken parts and bones, to slow boil for another 2-3 hours. Chop up some carrots, parsley, onions, and celery and one bay leaf. That's a chicken soup for fixing just about anything! (Because the bones are added, this can be referred to as chicken stock. If you don't use the bones, reduce the slow boiling time to half.)

If roasting a chicken, rosemary or garlic are great to season with, and other chopped herbs can be blended into the seasoning. Also, any vegetable stock can always include a medicinal tea.

Mayo and mustard: two useful condiments to enhance the flavor of foods. Do include them in your recipes. They are terrific carriers for dry, powdered herbs or tinctures. If you are using Dijon mustard, you can also use herbs that are not completely powdered, i.e., the barks or roots. Leaves and flowers should be powdered for the mayo—tarragon, rosemary, red clover, or alfalfa.

An alfalfa-mayo-nondairy butter, used as a dipping sauce for your cooked artichoke==a recipe for your liver and gallbladder.

Barbecue sauce, hot sauce, serious cayenne: It's best to put these aside for now given that they all include the nightshades.

Peanut butter and grape jelly: Think of peanut butter as your ally; what a friendly delivery system! Mix in a superfood, like spirulina or moringa, or your valued choice of a powdered plant or tincture. A ready-made, easy way to sustain plant benefits.

cake baking mixes
cookie baking mixes
waffle baking mixes
banana bread baking mixes
cornbread baking mixes
biscuit baking mixes
zucchini baking mixes
peanut butter baking mixes
chocolate chip cookie baking mixes
fudge baking mixes

Each one of these ready-made mixes is loaded with sweeteners, especially white sugar. Many people crave a sweet tooth after ingesting a meat; it's due to the sequence in the expansive-contractive continuum of foods. The mixes are usually overloaded on sweets and flavoring; reign in your tastebuds to what is closer to our original palate. These mixes can be augmented with tinctures, plant flours, or teas, including gymnema, "the sugar destroyer." Use just half of the baking mix, and then add 1 cup of a gluten-free flour to the bowl, along with ½ teaspoon of baking powder and 1 teaspoon of powdered gymnema or 8 to 10 drops of the tincture. (You can use gymnema tea as the water added to the mix.) You'll still be enjoying a favorite, old confection, which your digestive system will find easier to handle. As you transition away from overloading on tastebud stimulants, it's likely your nervous system will be less pumped, and your liver won't get a nightly workout eliminating sweets, thereby allowing for a more restful sleep. And, as a sweet tooth subsides, it becomes *easier to taste other foods again.*

George Ohsawa's List of Expansive to Contractive Foods

Expansive

- Drugs
- Alcohol
- Fruit juices
- Aromatic herb teas
- Tea/coffee
- Sugar
- Spices
- Fats and oils
- Tropical fruits
- Temperate fruits
- Sprouts/lettuce
- Fast-growing vegetables
- Tubers
- Bitter greens
- Sea vegetables
- Winter squashes
- Roots

- Nuts
- Beans
- Grains
- Fish
- Fowl
- Beef
- Eggs
- Tamari
- Miso
- Salt

Contractive (Colbin)

Dessert comes after dinner because sweetness is so tasty after a heavy meal of meat; your body is rebalancing itself. Familiarize yourself with this food continuum and recognize when your diet's been too weighted at one end or the other. (Pay attention to your cravings; they're a big clue about what your body needs next.) During the holidays, the season of sugar, ever notice how people "lose" themselves—because they've expanded too much? Likewise, a diet too heavy in nuts, beans, grains, and meats can make someone withdraw or perhaps "overthink." We need foods all along the continuum. And while some nutritional theories teach that you should eat "one of every food group" at every meal, my experience has been that it's okay to have "one of every food group" *in a day's time*. Meals can be simpler than what gourmet chefs prescribe; too many courses of too many flavors may sound like gastronomic merriment, yet the digestive tract is encumbered by having to sort it all out. The intestines, pancreas, and liver get busy with enzymes, hormone messengers, categorizing nutrients, and redirecting nutritional traffic. Here, the mothercrafting goal is to include enough medicinal herbs in your diet to rebalance your equilibrium, and in turn, transition to better food choices.

Triple-sugared breakfast cereals in super-king-sized boxes: The body wants protein for breakfast, and these packaged cereals contain manipulated carbohydrates. They're mega-dosed with sugar, high-fructose corn syrup, artificial sweeteners, maple syrup, agave, and honey. Allegedly to give you a boost to beginning your day, the body's endocrine system has its own waking-up scheme, and this sugar-shock can dysregulate how the body is pre-programmed to arise every morning. To begin with, you can fill your cereal bowl with ¾ of your cereal and make the other ¼ of the bowl a productive, nutritious fiber: oat bran or psyllium husks. Both the oat bran and psyllium husks help regulate your bowel movements, destress your colon, and add nutrients of their own. Their earthy flavors also help reorient your palate to a less excitable, sugar-laden taste.

Grains: Oats, rice, rye, buckwheat, cornmeal: The rules for cooking grains are straightforward. (1) Bring the liquid to a boil, (2) add in the grain and slow boil for 15 to 45 minutes, (3) stir several times when cooking. Instead of just boiling grains in water, boil them in a medicinal tea. Don't worry about making the tea very strong for a heavy dose of medicine; begin with a light tea, allowing your palate time to shift toward the reflavored grain as it becomes a regular part of your diet. As you detoxify and rebuild your core, your tastebuds will shift and welcome a stronger dose of tea. The grains are perfect for absorbing the liquid, with rice and quinoa especially good at puffing up. When adding treatment teas to your grains, sprinkle these same herbs on your chicken or fish, and toss some into your salad; your diet is closely mimicking the way our cavepeople ancestors practiced arcane, practical herbalism.

Coffee, expresso, black tea bags: When Western culture began drinking coffee and black tea in the 1600s, they were the only energy boosters around—humans had never felt a "kick up" like that before. Life was slower then, waking with the sun and sleeping with the moon. There wasn't the need for "fixes" to accommodate an agrarian-village lifestyle. A few sips of coffee gave the blacksmith the energy to finish the farmer's new harness for his oxen. A cup of black tea carried a mother farther afield, foraging for root vegetables while towing two little ones close behind. But the profound effect of racing to the New World expediated progress in our culture, values, duties, and responsibilities. Today, we live in rush hours keeping up with the Joneses, building careers, chasing social media, and bracing against office politics. This is an accelerated spin cycle of an adversarial, metropolitan society that warehouses people wanting to get more done. And product companies are always looking for the next "hot" ingredient for this society. Energy shots, stay-awake pills, sports drinks, and booster beverages of every size, shape, color, texture, and flavor are now found on supermarket shelves and in gas stations. The pharmaceutical industry willingly obliges with prescription stimulants and variations on a dextroamphetamine–amphetamine combinations. "Party pills" and "uppers" are socially accepted. This full-throttle operation of a hurry-up lifestyle has begat paid seminars on slowing down to smell the (virtual) roses. If the only way you can accomplish every item on your schedule is by revving up, then your body's telling you it's time to slow down. If you cannot keep up with your schedule now, try taking a step back. It's about making choices. There're culinary combinations that do provide energy, with long-term stamina as the end game. Likewise, there're food combinations and many good herbs that do help with relaxation. Coffee, expresso, and black tea served their purpose once…and it was a different purpose.

As you begin to slow down drinking coffee, expresso, or black tea, you can still add 2 to 8 drops from a tincture into each cup for your healing regimen.

"Nature does not hurry, yet everything is accomplished."

— Lao Tzu

Orange-aid/fruit punch/strawberry-kiwi/high vitamin-C juice boxes:
These juices are sweet and can be a nice, mid-day treat. Yet many are over laced with sweeteners, especially artificial ones (see Aspartame). Provisional fruit drinks can serve as "flavorings" when you cut them with a medicinal tea. Roughly speaking, green leaves and twigs have a green vegetable taste; think of the flavor spectrum of lettuce-peas-spinach. Roots and bark, roughly speaking, are on the flavor spectrum of wood-paper (remember putting a piece of white notebook paper on your tongue as a kid?). Time to experiment. A personal favorite is a splash of apple juice in a cup of pau d'arco tea. For a child, you may want a half-cup of juice poured into a half cup of tea. As one detoxifies, flavoring with fruit juices can be cut down.

The drinks are still "festive," and everyone is getting a delicious dose of something wholesome. Beginning daily with a juice-tea combo and then adding powdered herbs mixed in with some applesauce or non-dairy yogurt, provides good nutrition for the day.

There are certain herbs that have distinctive flavors on their own: rosemary, peppermint, licorice, black walnut hull, golden seal, sarsaparilla, sassafras, and garlic, to name a few. These are best suited for their own recipes (garlic and chicken, for example, or simply, a nice cup of peppermint tea).

Apples, blueberries, strawberries, bananas, broccoli, cauliflower:
These are wonderful fruits and vegetables. Consume them often. Today you can buy fresh or frozen strawberries every single week; *don't*. Remember, our bodies were designed for foraging and like variety more than our tastebuds do. Try something new, even if it's only once in a while. Papaya, artichoke, guava, red lettuce. Notice how your body regards this "pick me up" because each plant contains different, additional, nutritional constituents. You'll soon recognize when it feels like this one "just hit the spot...."

Frozen dinners of every genus, class, and brand: meat, chicken, fish, pizza, lasagna, pastas, chili, and plenty of side dishes: I believe Julia Child would have fancied this challenge: a freezer stuffed with prepared dishes and how-to-nourish-them-up. Maybe you were brought up eating frozen foods and they're still convenient. A single parent with a 50-hour-week job, two-hour commute, and three children doesn't have the time for gathering, making tinctures, simmering salves in a crock pot for three hours, and then making braised, butterfly pork chops, Roquefort-cheese-stuffed baked potatoes, and Bavarian crème pie. Recommending all of that equipment and uncustomary ingredients for a beginner just isn't prudent planning. Like other transitions you've made (remember going from childhood into adolescence?), there're bits and pieces to pick up, a zig here, a zag there, and then the momentum gets going. Likewise, as you explore healthier cooking, begin by grinding up an herb, like motherwort or saw palmetto, and mixing it with the mashed potatoes in your store-bought frozen dinner. (Yes, potatoes are a nightshade and better for some to leave them out; however, if they're in your freezer at this moment, make them work for you as they're a great delivery system for a ground-up root or tincture, etc.) Gravies and stews can always be perked up with teas, pizzas can be sprinkled with additional oregano combined with another ground green leaf, and lasagnas have those tasty layers that can be stuffed with a powdered bark or drops from a tincture. After dinner, have a nice cup of peppermint tea to soothe your digestive track.

Equipment

We need convenient nutritional delivery systems that easily fit into our cityscape of helter-skelter schedules and byzantine structures.

The three kitchen tools must-have to start:

- a small, electric coffee grinder
- a tea strainer
- a blender

Other kitchen tools as you go:

- tea kettle
- pots from small to large
- jars
- spatulas and long spoons
- mortar and pestle (or, to start: deep cup and hard spoon)
- measuring cups
- measuring spoons
- vegetable steamer
- mixing bowls from small to large
- juicer
- crock pot
- recipe file box or recipe notebook

Preparing and Seasoning Your Foods with Medicinal Herbs

Powdered herbs: You can purchase an herb in a powdered form, or you can grind it up yourself. If you already have a grinder for coffee beans, save that one for just coffee beans. Get a new grinder for your herbs. The idea here is to mix, blend, or sprinkle the medical vegetables into an already familiar recipe, accelerating the health boost in your customary foods. Remember, this forceful little machine grinds up hard coffee beans into a fine powder, so it's capable grinding up roots and nuts. Choices: do you use dried mullein leaves to make a cup of tea, or do you grind them up to add to a rice dish? Sprinkle them into some non-dairy yogurt to help with hay fever? These are easy choices. The more ways you utilize each plant, the more you'll learn about each delivery system and when to include which one.

Ground-up herbs can be sprinkled on casseroles, mixed into salads, blended into yogurts, or prepared with the seasonings for beef, chicken, fish, and casseroles.

Ground-up herbs can also be made into capsules (easily done by hand or with a small pill-making-machine found at a good, independent health food store or online).

Cooking versus raw: There is a value in eating raw foods in terms of how much "bang-for-your-buck" you get from an original source. The whole plant gives you a whole spectrum of vitamins and minerals which Mother Nature carefully calculated eons ago.

Even though heat/ovens/barbecuing/campfires/toasters will some-what de-nature the potency of a plant, a real benefit of cooking is that of softening the cellular walls in meats and plants. This makes them easier to digest for babies and people with compromised digestive systems, such as people getting older or who've survived cancer, etc. Being mindful of the nutrients lost in the cooking, you can make up for them in volume, i.e., additional servings of something nourishing or even adding in a few more medical vegetables related to a health issue throughout the day.

The Next-Step: Mothercrafting Your New Kitchen Cupboard

Non-Perishable Pantry Items

- brown rice, heirloom rice
- dry gluten-free pastas
- healthy cereals, granola, oatmeal, oat bran
- dried beans/legumes
- nuts: almonds, cashews, walnuts, pecans, pine
- nut butters, almond butter

- Liquid Aminos (gluten-free soy sauce)
- jams and jellies
- cooking oils: olive, avocado, sunflower, toasted sesame oil
- baking staples: whole wheat flour or gluten free flour, almond flour, almond meal
- honey, maple syrup, and stevia leaves
- baking powder, baking soda

Countertop produce

- beets
- hard/winter squash
- apples
- garlic
- onions
- bananas and other seasonal fruits

Refrigerator staples

- eggs
- "milk": soy, almond, coconut, cashew)
- "butter" (non-dairy)
- lemons and limes
- fruit juices
- dark breads: rye, barley, pumpernickel, flax, or oat; gluten-free breads, rolls, buns, wraps
- dairy-free cheeses, cheddar, parmesan, cream cheese
- kale, spinach, lettuce, red lettuce, sweet potatoes, celery, collards, winter squashes—butternut and acorn
- avocados, broccoli, cauliflower, onions, garlic
- tofu

Freezer

- Frozen fruits: strawberries, blueberries, mangos, blackberries, pineapple chunks

Household essentials

- veggie dishes
- ground beef
- chicken
- salmon, flounder, trout

Nice-to-haves

- olives, bottled salad dressings, pickles, sauerkraut
- freezer: (non-dairy) ice cream, sorbet

Kitchen-witching, old time teas, syrups, and tidbits for your daily remedies

> Ignore institutions; follow plants.

These recipes represent standard home meals as well as new ones developed in an urban herbalist's kitchen. The added flavors of whole roots, leaves, bark, berries, seeds, and flowers will enhance the recipe's earthiness, detoxify your body, rebalance your metabolism, encourage weight loss, boost your energy levels, and fit into your lifestyle. None of the ingredients on the Off-limits List are used here. Experimenting with cooking ingredients is one of the fun-est, grown-up things to try for the last 10,000 years. The dishes below have been knitted together for keeping away the adverse effects of disturbed, denatured foods and reinvigorating a modern person's menu. Initially, try each recipe, and then experiment with a pinch of this and a dash of that.

Before laptops and the internet, I was listening to a radio interview with a husband and wife photography team who wrote wonderful, easy-peasy, folksy cookbooks. They reminisced about driving the back roads in Appalachia, photographing wildflowers and sampling sweet apple pie, warm and fresh, baked in a cast iron stove. They drove through small towns, scouting effortless recipes and advice from real folks, who used real, every day ingredients. The wife explained, "No wonder they put Dr. Pepper into their meat loaf recipe. It's really just a brown, sugary syrup, and when the nearest supermarket is 40 miles away, you cook with whatever is available..." I've never forgotten both the sage wisdom and simplicity of that advice, nor the serendipitous versatility, too. A central idea to these mothercrafted recipes is that of taking proven medicinal herbs and mixing them into pre-existing recipes to enhance your health.

Adventures in Eating

Daily herbal teas: Put your tea into a thermos and sip it all day. You're adding more fluids to your body, much needed for health reasons, including constipation, skin enhancement, disposal of waste products, lubrication of joints, weight loss, blood building, and a fraternity of circulatory benefits. It's no oversight that Mother Nature tells us we're thirsty sooner than we're hungry; she wants us to drink more. For focusing on one specific health issue you're treating, you can also make a pot of a medicinal tea for cooking throughout the week. Anytime you need to add water to some dish, *add the herbal tea instead.**** Your rice will be more nutritious, your soups will have a tonic base, and your purees will be intensified.

***Make a big, pasta-pot of an herbal tea on a Sunday, and use it all week long in your recipes. For example, if winter is approaching, and you want to strengthen your family's immune system, then make a big pot of echinacea.

Use the echinacea tea as basis for a vegetable soup (cut up carrots, celery, green beans, onions, parsley, salt, and pepper; let simmer for 25-45 minutes, then steep for another 45 minutes). You can also drink the echinacea tea all as well as add it to other dishes. Add ¼ cup of the tea to a smoothie or add the tea to ½ glass of juice.

Making a pea soup or lentil soup or beans: Steep for 1-2 hours in the echinacea or another tea. Add more tea to the soaked peas, lentils, or beans to finish making each soup. Adjust the seasoning.

Rice: white, brown, basmati, Thai, black, bomba, jasmine, parboiled, sticky rice, red, long or short, or any other variety is particularly efficient for absorbing the virtues of whichever tea it is being boiled. This is a great delivery system for children or even pets.

Puree-whipping: always in an herbal tea: oatmeal, pasta, bananas, avocados, or other vegetables and grains.

For a chronic health issue, like breathing, include a variety of herbs in a variety of dishes: mullein, coltsfoot, elecampane, or elderberry. Add tincture drops to your morning smoothie, serve as a 10:00 a.m. cup of tea, pour into any sauce (substitute 1/8 cup of tea for any 1/8 cup of oil or milk or when lemon juice is called for, or for an egg white), use the tea as the water base for any puree, and substitute some tea for water when making pasta. Our bodies were designed for gathering, storing, recycling, and integrating nutrients from a variety of foods to be harnessed as fuel when needed.

As you learn the flavors, textures, and temperaments of the teas, and have factored together your health needs with chronobiology, the seasons, personal schedules, time of day, and wellness goals, you'll be better adept at planning ahead for meals. *(Who said we would never use those algebraic equations again?!!)*

Adding in an herbal tea, here and there

- In the stuffing for the Thanksgiving turkey, be it rice or breadcrumbs.

- I even mothercraft my cat's and dog's food with teas. Remember, in the wild, all animals nibble on plants. Cats are real carnivores, thereby leaving almost every cat with compromised kidneys by the time the cat reaches old age. I add tiny pieces of parsley, or parsley tea to my cat's food. Here is a plant just for cats and not for humans: crab grass. Cats love it, and it helps with the assimilation of food. Dandelion root tea benefits dogs. In addition to its nutrients, especially potassium, it is a great detoxifier. Blood cleansing is good for cholesterol and for the heart.

Herbs as side dishes: The same way carrots or asparagus can stand alone as side dishes, so can a number of herbs. Burdock is a frequent side dish in Japan. Begin experimenting with how to serve them.

The recipes presented in this book do illustrate how to nutritionally enhance what you're used to preparing. You can mix-and-match, scramble, condense, or elaborate in any direction your chef's imagination takes you. Yet the apothecary-practitioner-chef still needs to analyze the sum of the parts. If you add three cups of sugar to a cake, the value of mixing in a medicinal herb is lost because your body's busy filtering out the overload of glucose from that batter. You cannot drink alcohol all night, take an herb, and the next day feel fine. The idea is not "to mask" the partying or unhealthy food choices; the idea is to help preserve the body's health integrity, remain in homeostasis, prevent an illness from ensuing, and still enjoy an epicurean feast from Mother Nature's garden. **Apple sauce, yogurt, and mashed sweet potatoes are dandy carriers of nearly every offering in Mother Nature's pharmacopoeia.** Tasty and mushy, you can add in ½ teaspoon of a powdered or chopped herb, or ten drops from a tincture, or use tea as the base for apple sauce and sweet potatoes. What other dishes do you already have that are nice and mushy?

When I want to sweeten an herbal tea, I add a splash of apple juice or stevia tea, tea from the steeped stevia leaves, not the crystalized white powder sometimes sold in packets. I keep a bottle of the stevia tea in my refrigerator to add here-and-there at any time.

Quick Starts Roll Call:

- 1 part anise, ½ p. caraway, and ½ p. catnip==a good anti-colic or carminative tea.
- ½ part anise, 1 p. each thyme and horehound, into honey for a syrup==a cough remedy.
- 1 part catnip, ½ p. marjoram & pinch of saffron tea==measles remedy. Follow with a healing paste of cooked oatmeal, flax seed meal, and chopped plantain (Cook oatmeal in plantain tea.)
- Sweeten woody roots and bark teas with a splash of apple juice or cranberry juice.
- 1 part coltsfoot, ½ p. horehound, and ½ p. marshmallow, honey syrup==cough remedy.
- 1 part turmeric, ¼ p. ginger, ½ p. meadowsweet tea==antioxidant and joint support.
- 1 part cleavers, ¼ p. parsley, and ½ p. marshmallow==urinary and bladder issues.
- 1 part red clover, 1 p. burdock, 2 p. Oregon grape root==bronchial troubles, whooping cough, and viral infections tea.
- Sprinkle some fennel seeds on different, soft, warm dishes, i.e. oatmeal, lasagna, soups, fruit pies==the fennel will stimulate the colon to keep it moving.

Basil, sweet marjoram, summer savory, thyme, sage (and one or two green medicinal herbs): tie into a two-inch-square cheesecloth bag or small muslin bag. Infuse into your soup stock for 10-15 minutes. All herbs should be dried. Season to taste.

Add to chicken or turkey broth: sweet marjoram, sweet savory, sweet basil, chervil, thyme, tarragon, rosemary, chives, parsley (and one or two other green medicinal herbs) as an undried mixture. Season to taste.

A Wild Thyme in the City: Mothercrafted Recipes Readymade

10:00 a.m. Snacks

- Zip lock bag with 4-6 baby carrots and 15-20 raisins.
- Hummus with three small pieces of celery or bean chips.

Anytime yogurt

~ One container of dairy-free vanilla yogurt (optional: add in a combo of one Tbs of psyllium husks or oat bran, sliced peaches or sliced mangos; also: ¼ tsp of cat's claw, spirulina, or matcha tea or another powdered herb).

~ Vanilla coconut yogurt with sliced papaya==soothing support for an over-stressed, compromised, intestinal tract.

Good mood morning muffettes

- Mash two bananas in a bowl
- 1/3 cup maple syrup
- 1 cup of almond, coconut, or soy milk
- 2 eggs
- 1/8 teaspoon salt
- 2 tsp baking powder

- 2 tsp vanilla extract
- 1 cup non-dairy yogurt (almond, coconut, cashew, or soy)
- 1 Tbs cinnamon
- 3 cups of uncooked oatmeal (or, 2 ½ cups oatmeal and ½ cup of oat bran)
- 1 Tbs of ground St. John's wort

~ Combine all wet ingredients, then add in all dry ingredients.

~ Use little paper cupcake shells in the pan. Pour mixture into each cupcake shell.

~ Top with blueberries, cranberries, wineberries, sliced apples, or almond slices

~ Bake 350 degrees for 30 minutes.

Favorite, no-fail delivery systems for ingesting healthy herbs in a tasty way.

Yummy, Lumpy New England Apple Sauce

Moms & Dads, you can hide *anything* in applesauce. Here's a recipe I make every fall when New England is bursting with apples. It's also gentle on one's tummy, for someone with food allergies or even a pregnant woman.

- six big fresh apples (Cortland, McIntosh, or your favorite)
- ½ cup of honey
- 1 tsp cinnamon
- ½ tsp of ginger
- pinch of finely ground pink salt

~ Peel the apples, and cut into pieces. In a medium-size pot, bring 2 cups of water to a boil (may use an herbal tea here), and put the apple pieces and salt into the boiling water. Lower the flame, and let simmer for 20-25 minutes, or until mushy and lumpy. Use a potato masher to get out the big lumps. Then, add in the honey, cinnamon, and ginger, and simmer for another 10 minutes. Stir and turn off the flame. Let stand for an hour.

~ While you can eat it right from the stove, I've found little children really enjoy it when it's been chilled in the refrigerator for a few hours. Use as a side dish to any meal, as a treat, or put about 1 cup into a small bowl and add *any* powdered herb or tincture to it. The applesauce flavor is so vibrant, it masks the bitters or dry taste of barks and roots. By leaving it a little lumpy, it's even easier to disguise the added herbs. The best delivery system when children (or even us adults!) need to take another dose of something. (Roots, bark, and seeds work well when added in *after the applesauce is made, and you're ready to serve it.*) For one cup of chilled applesauce, add in ¼ tsp to ½ tsp of herb or 6 to 10 drops of tincture.

Electuaries 101

An electuary is a delivery method prepared by simply mixing dried, pow-dered herbs combined together with a sweetener, and a nut butter: peanut, almond, cashew, macadamia, or Brazil nut, and sometimes, a fruit pulp. They take the forms of cubes or bars. They can be molded into bite-sized portions. This is a modern-medieval remedy for 21st-century urbanites whose on-the-go lives are wrapped around computers, remote job sites, non-stop travel, and keeping up with the latest social media on the latest digital platform. Saving time is on everyone's list. Urban herbalists are carving lives out of skyscraper canyons and commuter rails while adapting helpful, verified remedies into their lives. In between this bustle, making these healthy snacks is one more way to show up for yourself. The fluid sweeteners can be honey, honey cream, maple syrup, maple cream, or agave nectar. Dry, powdered stevia leaves may also be used. A fruit paste binder is another option and can be made in a blender with a fluid sweet-ener and chopped prunes, dates, figs, raisins, dried cranberries, or apricots.

Merengue Bars! Merengue is a style of Latin Caribbean couple-dancing that is close, fast, and lots of fun. While tweaking this energy bar recipe to include moringa, I named them "merengue bars" because you'll have so much energy when you try one, you'll want to get up and dance!

- ¾ cup raw almond butter
- ½ cup honey
- ¼ tsp vanilla extract
- 1 Tbs coconut oil
- ½ cup unsalted, toasted sunflower seeds
- ¼ cup shredded coconut meat
- 1 cup almond flour
- ½ tsp non-dairy butter
- 1 Tbs moringa (or powdered herb of choice)
- Optional: chopped raisins or cranberries

~ In a large bowl, combine all moist ingredients: almond butter, honey, vanilla extract, coconut oil, and non-dairy butter. Mix well.

~ Add in dry ingredients: coconut meat, almond flour, moringa or powdered herb of choice. (optional: raisins or cranberries.) Mix well.

~ Into a buttered 8" by 8" pan, firmly press energy bar "dough." Pat down to ¾ inch across the pan, cover and freeze for 2 hours or more. About 10 minutes before serving, remove from freezer and cut into small squares. (You can also vary this by rolling the dough into small, bite-size balls and put each one into a square of an ice cube tray.) Dried herbs absorb moisture from a batter; depending on which herb used, you may need more honey, etc. For example, if you make one with dried mullein or coltsfoot for respiratory issues, add a little more honey (which may further help a sore throat). For a-detox-after-an-evening-of-partying, use gravel root/Joe Pye Weed and milk thistle (seeds). These are a little more "crunchy," which is fine, so add more almond butter. (Adding crunchy almond or crunchy peanut butter works well with finely chopped roots or seeds.) Lastly, add in ¼ tsp bee pollen for extra energy and a dose of amino acids, vitamins, and as a regional adaptogen. Like many a recipe, play with the ingredients. After they're made, put them into an airtight container and store in the refrigerator. They usually become a popular treat, so they don't last very long. These little cubes can be made quickly, and it's a great way to involve children in the process of taking care of themselves. (Who gets to lick the bowl?)

Chyavanprash. Do what Ayurvedic apothecaries have been doing for 5,000 years: put an entire electuary mixture into a jar of honey and spoon it by the dose or use it for a jam. (Add two Tbs of ghee to a 16-oz jar of honey.) Definitely, the world's first authentic, organic, plant-based multivitamin, superfood was Chyavanprash, the granddaddy of all Ayurvedic formulations. Considered a daily rejuvenator for energy, it is thought to be one of the oldest recorded botanical formulas in herbal medicine. (Indian families will have a personal Chyavanprash recipe handed down for generations.) Ayurvedic practitioners discovered combining herbs from different health categories resulted in support for aging and longevity. While the health food industry is selling various combinations of familiar Western fruits and Western vegetables, you can combine a group of powdered medical vegetables maximizing your nutritional boost and using it daily like "a treatment." Use a very good, local honey from a local bee keeper, and add to the jar one part each for each of the following lists.

Western, New Age Chyavanprash: alfalfa, astragulus, blessed thistle, chickweed, cleavers, coltsfoot, devil's claw, ginger, ginkgo, meadowsweet, milk thistle, nettles, Oregon grape root, rosehips, sarsaparilla, Siberian ginseng (eleuthero), yellowdock. (Add in dong quai and red raspberry for a women's blend. Add in saw palmetto and damiana for a men's blend.)

Detox blend: yellowdock, Oregon grape root, nettles, milk thistle, ginger, dandelion, cornsilk.

Respiratory blend: elecampane, amla, coltsfoot, holy basil, chicory, mullein, hyssop, bee pollen.

Prepare for Pregnancy blend: alfalfa, red raspberry, burdock, black haw, chamomile, ginger, nettle, cramp bark, slippery elm bark, and motherwort. **(Do not take this during pregnancy.)**

Men's Soldiering On blend: saw palmetto, schizandra berry, sarsaparilla, pau d'arco, hawthorn, nettles.

Laxative Colon Cleanse: fruit paste binder of prunes, figs, raisins, and honey, combined with cascara sagrada, black walnut hull, ginger, and meadowsweet.

Cosmic Smoothie

A delightful invention of the natural foods' movement, smoothies are a tasty way to enjoy your own, daily eupeptic.

How to Make a Cosmic Smoothie

Ingredients: Combine the fruits, veggies, "milk," and herbs of your choice, according to your taste and necessity. You don't have to add all these ingredients; pick your favorites, and try varying them daily. Rotating the ingredients helps because your body does need different things on different days. I never use the exact mixture two days in a row.

- 1 cup almond, cashew, soy, or coconut "milk." Excellent source of protein, good for lactose intolerance or hyperactivity. Add more "milk" as needed.

- ½ to 1 cup favorite combos of seasonal fruits:
  - blueberries, strawberries, banana
  - mangoes, coconuts
  - blackberries, banana
  - papaya, coconuts
  - cacao, wineberries or raspberries
- 4 Tablespoons plant protein powder (Choose a protein powder that DOES NOT CONTAIN an encyclopedia of vitamins, minerals, amino acids, and the latest "hot" ingredient. The nutrients will come from the herbs added to this mixture.)
- 1 teaspoon to 1 Tablespoon powdered herb.***

Optional: Add *one or two* of the following to fortify the nutritive value of your smoothie.

- ½ cup plain or vanilla yogurt; the friendly bacteria help your intestinal tract; it thickens the smoothie.
- ½ tsp of lemon juice; detoxifies and kills germs; breaks down fat.
- 1 tsp of lecithin; a fat emulsifier; promotes energy; helps repair damage to liver (especially by alcoholism).
- 1 tsp of oat bran; activates lowering cholesterol; gently moves and cleanses intestinal tract; food for nerve cells **or** 1 tsp of psyllium husks; good intestinal cleaner and stool softener.
- choose one: leaves of kale, spinach, parsley or sprouts

***Add up to **1 tsp or 10 tincture drops for each of (no more than) three additional ground herbs**. Like the gatherers who nibbled their way through the woods, a chronic health issue is helped by various plantlets throughout the day, each one targeting the same health issue. For example, you may add some mullein to your breakfast smoothie, steam and inhale rosemary and eucalyptus leaves to open your nasal passages in the late morning, drink some elecampane tea at lunch, sniff cedar oil in the afternoon, and end the day with a few detoxification, homemade capsules of burdock and milk thistle. Combine some nutrients, store some nutrients, recycle some nutrients, and deliver some nutrients, all day.

Nut milks, Cosmic Smoothies, and Courageous Juices

Raw Vegan Cashew Milk or Raw Vegan Cashew Crème

Cashew "milk"

- ½ cup raw cashew nuts
- 2 cups water (or chosen tea)
- 1 teaspoon of agave or honey or maple syrup
- ¼ tsp each of cinnamon and ginger

~ In a bowl, place cashews and add water (tea). Cover and let soak 4 hours to overnight.

~ Place soaked cashews into a blender. If needed, add additional ½ cup of water (or tea) and blend 1 minute until smooth. Add sweetener, cinnamon and ginger, and refrigerate in a glass jar.

Cashew crème

- 2 cups raw cashew nuts
- Enough water (or chosen tea) to just cover the cashews while soaking
- 2-3 tsp of agave or honey or maple syrup
- ¼ tsp each cinnamon and ginger

~ In a bowl, place cashew nuts and add water (tea). Cover and let soak 4 hours to overnight.

~ Place soaked cashews into a blender. Blend on a high speed 1-2 minutes until smooth. Add in sweetener, cinnamon and ginger, and refrigerate in a glass jar.

This version is thicker, almost like a nut butter. Both are good for top-ping granola, oatmeal, or your favorite cereal. (½-1 tsp of a root or bark, chopped or powdered, can be mixed into the granola or oatmeal.) The crème version is particularly good for combining with the root herbs.

If a root or bark herb is needed for one's diet, than beginning with a breakfast like this, and drinking the tea of the root herb all day is met-abolically efficient. Oatmeal is effective for settling down a restless or over-stimulated child.

Bee Welcome Smoothie

- 2 heaping Tbs of almond butter, cashew butter, or cashew crème
- 1 heaping Tbs of vanilla vegetable protein powder
- ½ Tsp hemp protein
- 1 cup of coconut milk
- ¼ cup of diced mango
- 1 banana
- 1 tsp bee pollen and 1 tsp honey
- 1 heaping teaspoon of your powdered, nutritional herb

~ In a blender, puree all ingredients together. Depending on which herb you added, you may want to adjust the amount of the added honey and diced mango.

Matcha Cha Cha Vanilla Smoothie

- 1 banana
- 4 Tbs of vanilla plant protein powder
- 1 tsp of powdered matcha or ¾ cup of matcha tea (If matcha tea is used, a second banana can be added to thicken the smoothie.)
- ½ tsp of vanilla
- 1 cup of almond or coconut milk
- 1 tsp of any other green leaf medicinal herb

- Optional: a second tsp of a medicinal herb. If optional herb is added, add ½ tsp of maple syrup.

~ This is a real energizer for beginning a day as well as a substitute meal.

Colon Comfort: Cucumber & Pineapple Breakfast Juice

~ In a blender, add together ¼ cup sliced cucumber, ½ cup diced pineapple, ½ cup marshmallow tea, 1/8 tsp turkey rhubarb, and ¼ tsp cascara sagrada. Blend until smooth.

Especially good to clear out old fecal matter, this helps cleanse the colon. It allows greater absorption through the intestinal villi, thereby enabling the villi to better absorb nutrients from the chyme. Feeling greater satisfaction after a meal, there are fewer cravings. When the body continues craving after a meal, it's a sign it's seeking minerals in order to rebalance itself (homeostasis).

Other Juicer Recipes

Cold & Flu
Carrot, mango, lemon, ginger, cleavers tea

Constipation
Apple, grapefruit, cucumber, ginger, triphala (powdered Ayurvedic herb combination)

Gastritis
Sweet potato, ginger, turmeric, apple, celery, mugwort tea

Bronchitis
Broccoli, cabbage, ginger, garlic, elecampane tea

Thyroid
Beet, carrots, pineapple, apple, 4 drops liquid kelp

Soups and Sauces

A Good Root Soup

You can start your spice-rack-herbalism-wellness-journey by making a good root soup. Soups are where our great-great-grandmothers simmered rich pots of bone broth enlivened with seasonings and cuttings from the forest and garden. Broths were more than delicious and loaded with complex, palliative mixes of natural ingredients.

It's perfect to begin adding herbal teas into canned soups starting today. After emptying the contents of the soup can into the pot on the stove, instead of filling it with water, fill it with a can of medicinal tea. (Begin with a tea of no more than two-three blended herbal teas.) The store-bought soup can may be high amounts of sodium ("fat free" equates to added salt for flavor); therefore, add at least one detoxification herb, like cleavers or alfalfa. What is great about a can of chicken noodle soup or mushroom soup as a base is that other ingredients add flavor. Granted, the flavor of the soup will change somewhat—but soups are traditionally the way to serve liquid vegetables.

Bone broth soups were standard fare for our ancestors because they were delicious, used all the ingredients these hunter-gatherers collected in a day, and helped with joints, skin, and vitality. To a pot of 6 cups of boiling water, you can add in the chicken carcass, neck, and some meat, as well as a combination of carrots, onions, garlic, kale, peas, broccoli, cauliflower, asparagus. You can also add in any combination of the following roots and bark: yellowdock, wild yam, white willow, turmeric, turkey rhubarb, slippery elm, pau d'arco, devil's claw, echinacea, or elecampane to start. By adding ginseng (panax) or Siberian ginseng (eleuthero), you are cooking a soup to invigorate and awaken. By adding valerian, you are cooking a soup for relaxing or going to sleep. You decide. Slow boil for 1-2 hours. Season with dashes of kelp and pepper.

If there is a flower or leaf herb whose nutrients you want to include, make them as teas beforehand, and add them in after the soup is finished boiling. Remember, they need less preparation time.

One more variation is to add in beef bones with some browned meat. Vary the herbs and seasonings to taste.

You may find a preference in either taste or results from chicken or beef. You decide. Remember to strain the bones out before you serve the soup.

Even as you introduce these new variations to your tastebuds, your body will already be receiving nourishment. The more detoxification from excipients, preservatives, and other additives, the more transitioning there'll be in your digestive tract, in turn leading to a healthier life.

Making Medicament Soups

Pea Soup

~ Boil 4-5 cups of water, and add 1 heaping Tbs of dried burdock root. Slow boil for 15-25 minutes.

~ Turn off the flame and let steep for 1 hour. (You can strain out the burdock root or leave it in. It can certainly be eaten when the soup is ready.) Soak 2 cups of dried peas in the burdock tea overnight.

~ The following day, add ½ tsp of dried onion or 1 Tbs of chopped onion with two sprigs thyme.

~ Nourishing and tasty, you can add ½ tsp of another root or bark herb. Let slow boil together for one-two hours on low-to-medium heat, stirring several times per hour.

~ Season when ready with onion, pepper, or celery salt.

Perfect White Bean Spring Tonic Soup

~ 2 cups of white beans, soak in just enough herbal tea to cover the beans overnight. (Root and bark teas herbs work well with white beans, enhancing the deep, earthiness of their flavor.)

~ Put in three cups of water/tea (use the same tea used for the overnight soak).

~ Add in any or all of the following:
  * ½ chopped onion
  * 2/3 cup chopped carrots
  * 3 sprigs of chopped parsley
  * ¼ cup of chopped celery
  * 2 sprigs of thyme
  * pinch of rosemary or pinch of celery salt

~ Bring to a boil and slow simmer for two-three hours.

~ Serve with a good dark, German rye bread or a gluten-free Ciabatta roll.

Chicken and Moringa Leaf Soup with Coconut Milk Ingredients

* 2 large chicken breasts, thinly sliced
* 3 to 4 cups fresh moringa leaves, stems removed or 2 heaping Tbs powdered moringa
* 1 small onion, chopped
* 3 cloves garlic, minced
* 1 two-inch piece of ginger, peeled and finely sliced
* zest from one lime
* 4 Tbs avocado oil
* 4 cups chicken bone broth (bone broth can be slow boiled in any herbal tea)

- 2 cups whole coconut milk
- 1-2 Tbs equal parts soy sauce and lime juice

~ Heat the avocado oil in a pot. Sauté the garlic, ginger, onion, and lime zests for one-two minutes. Add the chicken strips, browning on each side for 3-5 minutes. Pour in broth-tea. Bring to a boil, lower heat, cover, and simmer for 15-20 minutes or until the chicken is cooked through. Pour in the coconut milk, fold in the moringa, then add the soy sauce/lime juice. Stir. Bring to a boil, and then simmer for two minutes before turning off the heat. Avoid overcooking the moringa to reduce bitter flavor. Adjust seasoning to taste.

Celery Root & Parsnip Puree

- 2½ cups celery root, chopped
- 2½ cups parsnips, chopped (carrots can be substituted)
- pinch of pink salt or celery salt
- 4 Tbs ghee, olive oil, or vegan butter
- 1 tsp of powdered herb or ¼ cup chopped leaves or flowers or 1 Tbs ground up root, bark, or seed bark

~ In a large saucepan, add celery root, parsnips, and 2-3 cups of a leaf tea to cover the vegetables. Add pinch of salt, cover, and bring to a boil. Continue to slow simmer for 10-15 minutes or until the vegetables are tender enough to mash into a paste. Once cooked, remove from the stove top, remove the vegetables, and reserve the drained off the liquid. Place the pan back on the stove and add ghee, olive oil, or vegan butter. Place vegetables back in the saucepan with ½ cup of the reserved liquid and then mash them using a masher or firm whisk until smooth. Add more liquid until the puree's consistency is firm yet "creamy." Adjust seasonings.

Since a puree is so beneficial for the digestive system, bitter herbs go well with this easily digestible side dish. Keep in mind, the clearer your palate is, the less "inedible" you'll find a bitter. When bitters are tasted in the mouth, a message is sent to your gut to produce a digestive hormone. Bitters can support the liver in detoxification, increase the bile flow, and whet your appetite. Additionally, as your digestive tract heals, it will be easier to experiment with more plant varieties and seasoning combinations. The bitters include wormwood, rue, gentian (very strong), white horehound, hops, barberry, boldo, golden seal, chicory, hops, mugwort, blessed thistle, and parsley.

Black Beans

Black beans and brown rice do provide a hearty, balanced, nutritional meal. Vegan sour cream completes this timeless dish.

- 1 Tbs meadowsweet
- 2 ½ cups black beans

~ Bring four-five cups of water to a boil. Turn off the flame. Add meadowsweet and allow the infusion to stand for one hour. Strain out the meadowsweet. Put the black beans into the meadowsweet tea. Let stand for 4 hours to overnight. Bring the beans and meadowsweet to a slow boil and let simmer for 1-2 hours. Meadowsweet's anti-inflammatory properties and soothing of the intestinal tract are a good balance for the gas usually created by beans. For the brown rice, try making it in a different herbal tea to extend healing benefits. Top with vegan sour cream.

Ginger-Garlic Paste

- 1 3-inch peeled ginger root, thinly sliced
- 4 garlic cloves, thinly sliced
- ½ tsp of a different root herb
- 2 Tbs vegetable oil

- 1 Tbs of water (or a tea from the same root herb being added to the paste)

~ Combine all ingredients in a blender, and blend until smooth. This keeps for up to a week. Flavor meats, garnish veggies.

Salads & Bowls & Simply Veggies

Sweet Potato 101

- 1 long sweet potato, cut lengthwise into slices

~ Toast two slices in your toaster or toaster oven, 7-12 minutes.

Optional: use 4 drops of a tincture or ½ tsp powdered stalk or woody herb blended into one of these toppings:

- peanut butter spread
- 8-10 pieces of sliced banana, sprinkled with cinnamon or ginger
- almond butter, chia seeds, and blueberries
- refried black beans, fried egg, cilantro
- vegan ricotta, pear slices, honey
- vegan crème cheese, walnuts, honey

Arugula Pesto

- 1 cup of arugula
- ½ cup basil leaves
- ¼ cup chickweed or ¼ cup rue or ¼ cup other green leaf herb
- 2 garlic cloves, peeled and thinly sliced
- ¾ cup unsalted-roasted-finely chopped cashews
- ½ cup olive oil
- pink salt and pepper to taste
- ¼ cup non-dairy parmesan cheese, grated
- 1 Tbs lemon juice (optional)

~ In a blender, combine all ingredients until creamy. Pour over (gluten-free) pasta of choice and toss. Additional olive oil and grated parmesan may be added. Serve.

Impeccable Green Herb Creamy Pesto

- 1 cup chickpeas
- 1 cup basil
- 1 cup pine nuts (cashews may be substituted)
- 1 cup green leafy herb (or 20 tincture drops green leaf or flower herb)
- ¾ cup olive oil or avocado oil
- ½ cup tahini
- ½ cup nutritional yeast
- splash of lemon
- ¼ cup water (optional: ¼ cup herbal tea instead)

~ In a blender, combine all ingredients until creamy. Top with pine nuts (or chopped cashews) and drizzle of olive or avocado oil. Use it for spreading, dipping, or lavishing on your favorite pasta.

Creamy Dreamy Pasta

~ Put 2 cups of cashews into a bowl and add ¾ cup water/herbal tea. Let soak for two-four hours.

~ In frying pan, drizzle enough oil to cover the bottom of the pan. Chop up ½ medium onion and 2 cloves garlic. Toss into the pan and lightly brown for 10 minutes.

~ In a blender, add in the cashews, browned onions and garlic, salt and pepper to taste, and two sprigs of thyme. Mix well. (Add another ¼ cup of water/herbal tea as needed.)

~ Transfer sauce to a bowl and toss in 1 cup of chopped basil.

~ Cook your gluten-free pasta of choice, strain, and add to the sauce. Top with dairy-free parmesan cheese.

Nouveau Wok Stir-Fried Rice

- 3 cups rice, made in an herbal tea. The rice needs "to dry off" in the fridge for 4 hours or more before it's used in a stir-fry recipe.

~ Add enough oil to cover the bottom of wok.

You need a high smoke-point oil:
- Rice bran (490 degrees)
- Grapeseed (420 degrees)
- Peanut (450 degrees)
- Soybean (450 degrees)
- Vegetable (400-450 degrees)

~ Add in ¼ cup of chopped onions to the oil, and stir.

~ Add in one egg to scramble over the onion in the oil.

~ Add in two cloves of garlic, chopped.

~ Add in 1 tsp of mushroom powder or ¼ cup of finely chopped mushrooms.

~ Add ¼ cup chicken broth or herbal tea or herbal chicken broth.

~ Salt and pepper to taste.

~ Add ¼ cup steamed peas and carrots.

~ Add ½ tsp powdered medicinal herb.

~ Splash with sesame oil to taste.

~ Add in the rice, and sauté for 5-10 minutes until browned. Serve warm.

Forest Salad Greens

Mother Nature's original intention was for us to be wildcrafting our way through the woods, snacking on forest greens. Ingesting the whole plant allows your body to absorb, distribute, and store the nutrients for when needed. Any plant from which you can make an herbal tea may also be eaten as a vegetable; this is ancestral herbalism.

Lettuce. Let us consider the varieties: red leaf, green leaf, oak leaf, romaine, iceberg, Boston, bib, kale, arugula, spinach, radicchio, endives, frisee. (Good Housekeeping.com) The basis of every beckoning salad bar, this is your foundation for condiments, vegetables, garnish, or other delectable morsels. Green leafy vegetables fall along a spectrum of flavor and health value, so try each one. Understand too, their flavors behave differently depending on with what they are combined.

A few more greens: *water cress* (known for having "zero" calories), *early spring dandelion leaves, wood sorrel, lovage, nasturtium* (leaves and flowers, which make the salad pretty), *purslane,* and probably another 20–30 green leafy plants, depending on where you live. Get friendly with the local farmers at the farmer's markets and ask for advice. The more variety in your meals, the better for the body.

Non-Dairy Yogurt Chive Dip

- 1 cup non-dairy yogurt
- 1 tsp lemon juice
- 2 Tbs chives
- ½ tsp flower or leaf medicinal botanic

~ Use as a dip for veggies.

Blithe Spring Anti-inflammatory Salad

- 4 cups of spinach
- 1 cup of blueberries
- ½ cup of strawberries

- ¾ tsp powdered devil's claw (or 20 tincture drops)
- ¾ tsp powdered astragalus (or 20 tincture drops)
- 1 cup of toasted, sliced, (candied) almonds
- ½ avocado
- avocado oil-based dressing

Relaxed Kale Salad with Cranberries and Pecans

- ½ cup honey
- 1 Tbs Dijon mustard
- ½ tsp fresh lemon juice
- 1 tsp lemon zest
- ¾ cup olive oil
- ¼ cup radishes, sliced
- ¾ cup dried cranberries
- ¾ cup pecan halves, toasted
- 5 cups fresh kale, chopped
- ½ cup fresh green leaf medicinal herb (or 20 drops of herbal tincture)
- 1 cup vegan feta or another cheese

~ In a bowl, whisk together honey, mustard, lemon juice, lemon zest, and olive oil. In a larger bowl, combine, kale, radishes, cranberries, and pecans. Drizzle the larger bowl with dressing, and sprinkle with cheese.

Bowls are big now, probably because they have just the right amount of convenience and ingredients. The core recipes combine a protein, vegetables, and a flavor. Sauce over a base like greens, quinoa, or rice.

Quinoa-Taco Bowl

- 1 cup cooked quinoa (or barley or bulgar may be substituted)
- ¼ cup chopped, cilantro
- 2 Tbs lime juice
- 2 tsp extra-virgin olive oil (or avocado oil when using avocado)
- 1 cup chopped escarole
- ½ cup of green leafy herb (or 20 drops of herbal tincture)
- 1 scallion, thinly sliced
- 1½ cups non-dairy yogurt (sauce), divided (choice of adding pinch: dill, cilantro, mint, parsley, or other left over herbs)
- ½ cup black beans,
- ½ avocado, thinly sliced
- non-dairy cheese, cheddar or your choice

~ Combine quinoa, cilantro, lime juice, and oil in bowl and toss to coat; season with salt and pepper.

~ Toss escarole, scallions, green leafy herb (tincture), and half of sauce to coat.

~ Divide between serving bowls and top with quinoa mixture, beans, and avocado. Crumble non-dairy cheese on top. Pour rest of dressing on top.

Cranberry Quinoa Bowl

- 2 cups cooked quinoa (in herbal tea)
- ½ cup dried cranberries
- ¼ cup sliced scallions
- ½ cup sliced almonds
- 2 sprigs of parsley, chopped.
- 3 Tbs sunflower oil
- 2 Tbs maple syrup
- ¼ tsp of crushed garlic

- ½ tsp of powdered green herb or 1/8 cup of fresh green herb leaves or 20 drops of tincture

~ Toss all the ingredients together in a large bowl. Wonderful as a side salad or a midday snack.

Far East Bowl

- 1 cup cooked brown rice (in herbal tea)
- 3 cups salad greens (Experiment with different kinds of lettuce, kale, and herbal greens. For example, if using red lettuce, try adding asparagus.)
- 1 block firm tofu (4" x 4")
- 1 carrot
- 2 cups veggies (mushrooms, asparagus & zucchini)
- 1 sweet potato
- 1/2 cup salad dressing of choice
- Sunflower or avocado oil for skillet
- 1 avocado
- 20 drops of a tincture

~ Cook rice. Chop veggies and sweet potato, grate carrot. Make crispy tofu.*** Set aside.

~ Sautee veggies in an oiled skillet for 8-10 minutes.

~ Roast sweet potato at 350 F for 15-20 minutes.

~ Divide the rice, ingredients, and tincture into bowls. Top with crispy tofu and sliced avocado. Drizzle with dressing.

***Crispy tofu

~ *Pat dry as much as possible. Toss tofu in 1 Tbs oil, ½ tsp tamari or soy sauce, and 1 Tbs cornstarch or arrowroot starch. The starch makes the edges extra crispy. Spread prepared tofu on a cookie sheet, even if it fell apart when you tossed it. Bake at 275 F for 25 minutes.*

Auntie Flame's Turmeric, Chicken, and Kale Rice Bowl

- 1 cup of brown rice
- 2½ cups of water (root or bark tea)
- 6 Tbs olive oil
- 1½ cups of chopped kale
- 2 chopped cloves of garlic
- ½ cup chickpeas
- 1 pound of boneless, skinned chicken breasts
- 2 tsp of turmeric
- ¼ tsp celery salt
- 1 sliced avocado
- ¼ cup dry, roasted, unsalted sunflower seeds

~ Cook rice in herbal tea. While rice cooks, put skinned chicken breasts in baking dish at 300 degrees. Cook for 35-40 minutes.

~ In a pan over a low flame, add 3 Tbs olive oil with the garlic. Stir for 2-3 minutes, then add chopped kale and stir for 2-3 minutes. Add chickpeas, and transfer to a bowl.

~ When chicken is done, toss it with turmeric and celery salt. Then, in the same pan in which the kale and chickpeas were cooked, add in 3 more Tbs olive oil and brown the chicken on each side for 10-12 minutes.

~ Slice the chicken, and layer your bowls with rice, kale, chickpeas, sliced chicken, and sliced avocado. Sprinkle with sunflower seeds.

Brussel Sprouts Parquet

- 6 Brussel sprouts, sliced
- 1 tsp lemon zest and 1 tsp lemon juice
- 2 Tbs olive oil
- 1 heaping tsp Dijon mustard
- 2 tsp gluten free teriyaki sauce

- ¼ cup grated non-dairy parmesan cheese
- ¼ cup chopped walnuts or chopped Brazil nuts
- ¼ teaspoon powdered, green leaf herb
- celery salt and pepper

~ Place shredded Brussel sprouts in a bowl; zest the lemon over the sprouts. In another bowl, mix Dijon mustard, olive oil, gluten-free teriyaki sauce, lemon juice, powdered herb, celery salt and pepper. Pour mixture over the sprouts and toss. Add nuts and parmesan to slaw and toss again before serving.

Garlic Vegan-Parmesan Broccoli or Brussel Sprouts

~ Add olive oil to pan bottom or on a cookie sheet. Place 10 Brussel sprouts, halved, or 1 ½ cups broccoli florets, chopped, in pan or on sheet.

~ Mix together ¼ teaspoon celery salt, ¼ teaspoon garlic powder or minced garlic, and ½ teaspoon of powdered or crushed leaf or flowered herb. Sprinkle topping mix on broccoli florets or Brussel sprouts. Top with vegan parmesan cheese (to taste).

~ Bake 400 F degrees for 4-6 minutes.

Zucchini Fries

- Two zucchinis sliced lengthwise
- 1 cup gluten-free breadcrumbs, panko breadcrumbs, gluten-free matzo meal, or crushed blue tortilla chips
- 1 tsp garlic powder
- 1 ½ tsp minced garlic
- 1 tsp dried basil
- ½ tsp of powdered herb
- ½ tsp pink salt
- 2 eggs

~ Mix batter ingredients together. Dip zucchini slices into the batter, then place them on a lined cookie sheet. Bake at 425 degrees for 20 minutes.

Sauteed Kale

- 4 Tbs olive oil
- splash of water/tea
- 2 tsp garlic, minced
- 8 cups of lacinato or curly kale, destemmed and chopped
- ¼ tsp celery salt
- ¼ tsp black pepper
- 2 Tbs of herbal flower, stem, or leaf, chopped.
- non-dairy butter to taste

~ Pre-heat a large sauté pan for 1 minute. Add in olive oil and kale. Stir for 2-4 minutes, letting kale wilt. Once wilted, add splash of water/tea and non-dairy butter to taste. Add in garlic and herb, stir for two minutes or until water reduced. Remove from heat and add in celery salt and pepper.

Arugula with Peaches and (Non-Dairy) Cheddar

~ On a rimmed baking sheet, toast ¼ cup pecans at 350 degrees, tossing once, 4-6 minutes; let cool, then chop. Toss 6-8 cups chopped arugula, 1-2 sliced peaches, 2 ounces (non-dairy) sharp white cheddar (cut into chunks), and pecans. Top with dressing of your choice. Sprinkle one teaspoon of the dried herb across your salad or 10 drops of a tincture. Toss well.

Sweet Potato and Carrot Tzimmes

I always tell my students that when they make a new friend, especially from another culture, invite yourself over for dinner. Chances are you'll be introduced to some new, scrumptious dish of food. This recipe is from the Ashkenazi Jews.

- 4 Tsp olive oil
- 2 cups diced carrots
- 3 medium-large sweet potatoes, peeled
- 8 pitted prunes, halved
- ½ cup dried apricots, chopped
- 1 small yellow onion, chopped
- ½ cup orange juice
- ½ cup raisins
- ½ teaspoon of cinnamon
- ¼ tsp cardamom or nutmeg
- ½ tsp ginger
- 1 cup brown sugar
- 1 Tsp finely ground medicinal herb, bark or root or 10 drops of tincture, bark or root***
- 1¾ - 2 cups water/herbal tea

***If 10 drops of tincture used, then only add 1 ¾ cup water.
***If 1 Tsp finely ground herb used, then add 2 cups of water.

~ In a large pot, heat the oil on medium-high. Add the onion and cook for 8-10 minutes. Add water and sweet potatoes. Bring the mixture to a slow boil and simmer. Cover and cook 35-45 minutes. Add in the rest of the ingredients and continue slow boil for another 10-15 minutes or until the sweet potatoes are tender. Uncover the pot and continue simmering another 5-10 minutes, or until it's thickened. Remove from stove. About 8 servings. Add salt and pepper to taste.

Five Easy Salad Dressings

Honey/Mustard Dressing

~ Blend: 3 Tbs extra-virgin olive oil, 2 Tbs freshly squeezed lemon juice, 1½ teaspoons of honey.

~ Add in: 2 Tbs Dijon mustard, ½ clove of garlic, grated or minced, pinch of finely ground pink Himalayan salt.

Creamy Herb Dressing

~ Blend: ½ cup buttermilk or unsweetened almond milk, ¼ cup mayonnaise.

~ Add in: 2 Tbs freshly chopped parsley, dill, chives, and one part of a preferred green leaf herb, dash of pepper.

Grand Lemon-Garlic Dressing

~ Blend: 1/3 cup olive oil, 2 Tbs fresh lemon juice.

~ Add in: ½ clove of garlic, grated or minced, pinch of pink Himalayan salt, dash of pepper.

Tahini-Garlic Dressing

~ Blend together ¼ cup tahini (creamy sesame paste) and ½ cup water or herbal tea.

~ Add in ¼ tsp of garlic clove or minced garlic and 1 tsp lemon.

Tahini-Orange Dressing

~ Blend together: 4 Tbs tahini with ½ cup water or herbal tea, 1 medium orange, peeled and seeded, ½ tsp mustard-dry or Dijon, and 2 tsp honey

~ Season to taste.

Baked Dishes

Black Walnut (Juglans nigra)

The drupes are harvested in the fall, dehulled, and dried to allow the nut meat to cure for consumption. Black walnuts contain the highest concentration of juglone in the nut hulls, roots, and leaves of any plant. The juglone serves as an herbicide and is a hot spot of anti-tumor research re: inhibiting the proliferation of malignant tumor cells. This tree has numerous uses: nutritional, medicinal, dye, structural/decorative, antibacterial, and herbicide. Furthermore, these nuts are a great source of mood-relaxing serotonin, always a benefit for a busy life.

Chicken Quiche with Black Walnuts

- 1 cup finely chopped chicken
- 2 cups (non-dairy) Swiss cheese, grated
- ¼ cup yellow onion, chopped
- 3 eggs, beaten
- ½ tsp Dijon mustard
- celery salt and pepper to taste
- 1 cup (preferred non-dairy) milk/half and half
- 1 cup chopped black walnuts
- 1 baked 9-inch gluten-free pie crust

~ **Directions:** Preheat oven to 325 degrees. Toss chicken, cheese, onion, and ½ cup black walnuts. Place in prebaked gluten-free pie shell. Beat the eggs with (non-dairy) milk/half and half, mustard, celery salt, and pepper and gently pour over the chicken/cheese mixture in the pie shell until the liquid reaches the edge of the crust. Sprinkle with the remaining black walnuts. Bake in the center of oven for 45 minutes or until top is lightly browned and filling is set. Serves 6-8.

Rice Balls

~ Bring 6 cups of medicinal tea to a boil, add in 4 cups of brown rice, and let simmer for 25 minutes. After rice is cooked, combine with: 3 eggs, 3 sliced garlic cloves, ½ cup grated (non-dairy) parmesan cheese, ½ cup parsley, salt and pepper to taste (optional). Taking a handful of the rice mixture, shape it into a ball. Then, take two fingers and push down into the center of each ball. Stuff a 1-inch "cube" of (non-dairy) cheese into the center of each ball. Roll each ball into another egg batter and sprinkle on gluten-free breadcrumbs. Gently put each ball into a pot of boiling water and cook for 2-3 minutes. Remove from water and put on a tray. Serve as a side, main dish or appetizer. Can be dipped into (no nightshade) marinara sauce. The rice balls can also be frozen and served later.

No Nightshades Marinara Sauce

- 4 Tbs olive oil
- 2 yellow onions chopped (no more than 2 cups)
- 3 minced garlic cloves
- 2 tsp dried basil
- 2 tsp dried oregano
- ½ tsp dried medicinal herb (leaves or flowers)
- 1 pound of carrots, chopped
- 1 medium beet, chopped
- 1 ½ cup of herbal tea
- ½ teaspoon of celery salt
- (optional: 1 Tbs of lemon juice or ¼ cup mushrooms, chopped).

~ In a deep pan, heat oil on low to medium, sauté onions for four minutes. Add in garlic, basil, and medicinal herbs, and stir for two minutes. Add in herbal tea, carrots, beets, and celery salt (optional: add in mushrooms). Simmer for 20 minutes or until tender. Pour contents into a blender (optional: add in lemon juice). Blend for 2-3 minutes or until smooth. This can be stored in a jar, in the refrigerator.

Store-bought Marinara Sauce #2

~ For a store-bought marina sauce, ½-1 cup of an herbal tea can be stirred in, or ½ - 2 tsp of a powdered herb depending on the quantity and thickness of the sauce.

Incredible Almond Oil - Brown Rice Sauce

- 4 cups of almond oil
- ½ cup Liquid Aminos
- 1 Tbs nutritional yeast flakes
- ½ tsp powered kelp
- ½ tsp powered green, medicinal herb
- ½ tsp celery salt
- 1 tsp minced garlic
- ½ tsp lemon juice
- 1 Tbs lecithin

~ Combine all ingredients in a blender. Pour into a serving bowl with a ladle (the mixture tends to settle after a few minutes, so keep stirring during mealtime). Prepare three cups of brown rice. (Brown rice should be boiled in medicinal herb tea.) Allow guests to ladle the almond sauce over their rice.

Spinach Tortillas

Tortillas are so versatile and can be used for breakfast, lunch, dinner, and even deserts! Here's an easy recipe for a gluten-free, spinach tortilla for your favorite filling:

~ Combine well in a blender: 1 cup of chickpea flour (also called garbanzo bean flour); ½ cup tapioca flour/starch; 2 cups of baby spinach; 1 cup of medicinal tea (add up to 1/8 more cup of medicinal tea depending on the thinness and/or largeness of the tortilla you want).

~ Pour between ¼ cup to 1/3 cup of batter into a non-stick skillet on a low-medium flame and cook for up to 2 minutes on each side.

Understand that these tortillas will not be thin like traditional tortillas, yet can be used the same way and do deliver twice the nutritional value. Season to taste.

~ Fillings can include rice, beans, chicken, ground beef, or veggie combos. ¡Hay many tasty posibilidades! Into your fillings is where you may add another medicinal herb—either healthy doses of cilantro or parsley, or ¼ teaspoon of a powdered herb mixed into the ground beef.

Main Dishes:
Chicken and Fish, and a word about meats

Meats do well being stewed in herbal teas, with tinctures added to gravies, and with powdered herbs mixed into spice blends.

Lime Broiled Chicken with Avocado and Corn

Lime Barbecue Sauce

- ½ cup corn oil, 2 tsp dried tarragon, ¼ cup lime juice, 1 Tbs lime zest, 2 Tbs chopped onions, ½ tsp chopped parsley, 1 tsp ground green herb or 1 tsp powdered root or bark.
- Other ingredients: 6 boneless chicken breasts, 2 husks of cooked corn, 2 avocados.

~ Preheat oven to 375 degrees. Combine all ingredients for Lime Barbecue Sauce. Marinate the chicken breasts in the sauce for 2-3 hours before baking. Place chicken in baking pan, and cook until tender (1 ¼ to 1 ½ hours). Top with slices of avocado and corn (Optional: place chicken breasts on beds of salad greens and then top with avocado and corn.) Season to taste.

Grilled Lemon-Rosemary Catfish

- 4 Tbs olive or sunflower oil, 2 tsp fresh rosemary leaves, 1 tsp lemon juice, ¼ tsp garlic powder, ½ tsp ground medicinal herb, 4 catfish fillets, celery salt and pepper, (optional: rosemary sprigs).

~ Coat grill with olive or sunflower oil and pre-heat to medium heat.

~ In a small saucepan, heat 4 Tbs olive or sunflower oil with lemon juice, rosemary leaves, garlic powder, and medicinal herb over medium heat for 1 minute.

~ Brush one side of each fillet with mixture. Season with celery salt and pepper. Grill fillets, 4-5 minutes. Turn fillets, brush with the rest of the mixture, and grill another 4-5 minutes, or until fish is tender. (Optional: garnish with rosemary sprigs.)

Aspiring Salmon

- ¼ cup Liquid Aminos, ¼ cup pineapple juice, 1 tsp ginger powder or 2 tsp minced ginger, 2 cloves garlic minced, 1/8 cup of water of herbal tea, 4 salmon fillets, 1 Tbs sesame seeds, olive oil or avocado oil to coat grill. (Optional: 16 drops herb tincture.)

~ In a bowl, whisk together Liquid Aminos, pineapple juice, ginger, garlic, and water/tea. Pour into a baking dish and marinate the salmon on both sides. Cover and refrigerate for 30 minutes.

~ Coat grill with oil and preheat to medium-high heat. Grill fillets for 5-6 minutes per side until tender. Remove from grill and place on platter. Sprinkle with sesame seeds. (Optional: put 4 drops of tincture on each fillet before serving.)

Artichoke-Parmesan Tilapia

- Four tilapia fillets, 4 Tbs olive oil, 2 tsp garlic, ½ tsp thyme, pepper to taste, 1 cup gluten free bread crumbs, 6 artichoke hearts (drained and finely chopped), 3 Tbs non-dairy parmesan grated, 1 Tbs fresh parsley, chopped. (Optional: ½ tsp medicinal herb powdered)

~ Preheat oven to 375 F. Coat baking pan with olive oil. Place fillets in baking pan and brush with oil. Mix together garlic, thyme, pepper (and optional medicinal herb). Sprinkle over fillets. In a bowl, combine bread crumbs, artichoke hearts and parmesan and spoon over fillets. Bake 20-25 minutes. Serve with parsley on a platter.

Roasted Chicken with Sesame Glaze

- 2 Tbs minced, fresh ginger
- 3 Tbs toasted, sesame oil
- 2 tsp gluten-free tamari or Liquid Aminos
- ½ tsp ground fennel seeds
- ½ tsp root or bark medicinal herb
- ¼ cup of root or bark medicinal tea
- 1 - 1 ½ pound of skin-on chicken thighs, drumsticks, or breasts
- 2 tsp sesame seeds
- 2 scallions, sliced
- dash of nutmeg

~ Heat chicken in oven at 350 degrees for 45-55 minutes.

~ Heat a small saucepan over a medium heat. Add in ginger and sesame oil, and then sauté the ginger for about a minute. Add in gluten-free tamari or Liquid Aminos, and simmer while the liquid reduces to ¼, 5 to 7 minutes. Add in fennel seeds, medicinal herb, medicinal herb tea, scallions, and dash of nutmeg. Let simmer for 10 minutes.

~ Add chicken to pan, and let cook for 6-8 minutes, a golden brown skin and well saturated.

~ Place chicken back in the oven for another 25-30 minutes. Sprinkle with sesame seeds when removed from oven.

Hor D'oeuvre

English Tea Sammie Bites

~ Finely chop and mix 1 Tbs chives and dill into ½ cup lightly whipped cream cheese. Spread onto thin cucumber slices. (Optional: add ¼ tsp powdered herb to mix.)

Deserved Desserts

Banana Peanut Butter Bars

- 2 bananas
- ¼ sunflower oil or coconut oil
- 1/3 cup honey or agave
- ½ cup crunchy peanut butter
- 1 cup oat flour
- 1 tsp baking powder
- ½ cup dark chocolate chips
- 2 tsp powdered medicinal herb

~ Combine all wet ingredients. Mix in oat flour, baking powder, powdered herb, and chocolate chips. Bake in pan at 325 degrees for about 20-25 minutes. Let cool, and then slice into bars. (Delicious when refrigerated after baking.)

Better Breakfast Cookies

- 1 cup almond flour or coconut flour
- 1/3 cup vanilla almond milk or coconut milk
- ¼ cup chopped pecans
- 1 cup chopped dates
- 1 tsp vanilla
- 2 Tbs dairy-free butter or coconut oil
- 1 tsp powdered Matcha (or other herb)

~ Combine wet ingredients, then add in dry ingredients. Drop cookie dough by the heaping tsp onto buttered cookie dough sheet.

~ Bake at 300 degrees, 12-16 minutes.

For the occasional sweet-tooth splurge, you can put a candle on anything and call it a "birthday cake."

Mum's Rosemary Pineapple Cake

- 2 cups gluten-free flour
- 1½ cups raw sugar (or one cup of honey; if honey is used instead of sugar, add ½ cup more flour & ½ tsp of baking powder)
- 1 cup of chopped pecans
- 1 cup chopped pineapple (save the juice for the frosting)
- 2 Tbs of fresh, finely chopped rosemary or 1 Tsp of powdered rosemary
- ½ tsp baking soda
- ¼ tsp of pink Himalaya salt
- 2 tsp of vanilla
- 2 eggs

~ Heat oven to 350 degrees. Butter cake pan with non-dairy butter. Blend together all wet ingredients. Gradually mix in all dry ingredients. Bake for 40 minutes or until golden brown.

Frosting:

- 8 ounces of non-dairy cream cheese
- ½ cup non-dairy butter
- 1 cup powdered sugar
- 2 teaspoons of vanilla
- saved pineapple juice

~ Put all ingredients in a blender and whip for 2 minutes. Frost the cooled-down Rosemary Pineapple Cake.

Zucchini Sesame Chocolate Cake

- 2 cups of gluten-free flour (almond flour or other flour)
- ¼ cup almond meal
- ¼ cup toasted sunflower seeds
- ½ teaspoon baking soda
- ½ teaspoon baking powder
- ½ teaspoon of pink salt
- 1 cup of honey
- ¼ cup coconut oil
- ½ cup chocolate chips
- ¼ cup water or herbal tea
- 1 teaspoon of vanilla
- 1 teaspoon of ginger
- ½ teaspoon of nutmeg
- 2 cups of grated zucchini
- 1 teaspoon finely ground, medicinal herb

~ Heat oven to 350 degrees. Butter your cake pan with non-dairy butter. Blend together all wet ingredients. Gradually mix in all dry ingredients. Bake for 40 minutes or until golden brown.

Cosmic Jamaican Banana-Nut Bread

A while ago when I was finishing my undergraduate degree and first learning herbal medicine, my friend talked me into a college-student's-kaleidoscope vacation in Negril, Jamaica. We never worried about where the boys were; we were girls who just wanted to have fun. When we landed (with Reggae music lilting out of every door and Bob Marley's picture in every shoppe), we found a serene, tropical island, flowers perfuming the air, and many happy, welcoming people. For nearly a month on this Caribbean island, our days were comprised of slow walks on chalk-white roads and sunning and swimming on sandy white beaches. Our evenings were filled with dancing and delicious banana daiquiris. Lots of American kids coming down, and our paradise was complete. Here's the recipe I created using delicious island ingredients including bananas, walnuts, and ganja:

- ½ cup butter (non-dairy butter, optional)
- ½ cup honey
- 2 eggs
- 1¾ cups of flour (gluten-free, almond, or coconut)
- 1 tsp baking powder
- ½ tsp baking soda
- 1 cup mashed bananas
- ¾ cup chopped walnuts
- ¾ cup ground mary jane

~ Cream together non-dairy butter, honey, and eggs. Sift together dry ingredients and combine with batter. Pour into a buttered, baking pan. Bake at 350 degrees for 45 minutes. Cool on rack. Enjoy. ☺

Pumpkin Tea Bread

- 2 ¼ cups cooked pumpkin
- 3 eggs

- ¾ cups apple sauce (See Yummy, Lumpy New England Apple Sauce)
- ½ tsp baking soda
- 1¼ tsp baking powder
- 1 tsp vanilla
- 2 cups sugar
- 3 cups gluten free flour
- 1 tsp each cinnamon, ginger
- ¼ tsp cardamom
- ¼ tsp pink Himalaya salt
- (optional: ¾ cup ground mary jane)

~ Grease two loaf pans.

~ Mix together moist ingredients, then mix in dry ingredients. Pour into pans. Bake 65-75 minutes at 350 F. Fun to serve with non-dairy butter or non-dairy cream cheese.

After delivering a lecture to the staff at a Whole Foods in Manhattan, I met a nice 65-year-old man in the aisle of the supplement department. He'd never bought a vitamin before, and wasn't sure how to shop. I showed him two different multivitamins, and he asked if he should buy them both. I asked him why he would do that, He said, "To be more healthy." I told him to choose one multi, and then to get the herb Saw Palmetto, explaining what an ally it is to an older man for supporting his prostate. He thanked me and even waved good bye.

I hope I have managed to put some questions and fears to rest by demystifying how to use herbs and how to apply them to your own health needs. Your body, your questions, the back and forth of the cultural landscape, an introduction to the materia medica, mothercrafting how-tos, and your kitchen cupboard. You've got this. And now you are ready to begin, even in the dollar store...

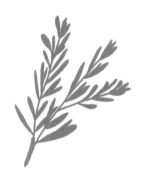
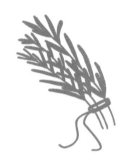

List of Works Cited

Arthritis. Dr. Michael T. Murray. Prima Health, 1994.

Better Health with Culinary Herbs. Ben Charles Harris, 1952.

Brief Guide to Biology. David Krogh, 2007.

Culpepper's Complete Herbal & English Physician. 1653.

Death by Medicine. Gary Null, PhD, 2010.

Disease Prevention and Treatment Life Extension. Sixth Edition, 2018.

Early American Herb Recipes. Alice Cooke Brown, 1966.

Food and Healing. Anne Marie Colbin, 1986.

Gerard's Materia Medica. 1633.

The Green Pharmacy Herbal Handbook. Dr. James Duke, 2000.

Health Knowledge. Dr. J. L. Corish, 1927.

The Herbal Handbook. David Hoffman, 1987.

Herbal Healing for Women. Rosemary Gladstar, 1993.

"Herbalgram," *The Journal of the American Botanical Council.* Mark Blumenthal, Founder.

Herbs for the Kitchen. Irma Goodrich Mazza, 1939.

Himalaya, USA Materia Medica. 2014.

Indian Herbalogy of North America. Alma R. Hutchens, 1991.

Journal of the National Medical Association, Vol. 85, No. 2. *The Flexner Report and Black Academic Medicine: An Assignment of Place.* Susan Hunt, EdD

The Lost Language of Plants. Stephen Harrod Buhner, 2002.

My House is Killing Me! Jeffrey May, 2001.

Nutrition for Healthy Living. Wendy Schiff, 2009.

Physician's Manual of Therapeutics. Parke, Davis & Company, 1901.

Prescription for Dietary Wellness. Phyllis A. Balch and James F. Balch, 1992.

Raw Food Real World. Matthew Kenney and Sarma Melngailis, 2005.

Ridgecrest Herbal's Almanac. 2022.

Staying Healthy with Nutrition. Elson M. Haas, MD, 1992.

Taber's Cyclopedic Medical Dictionary. Revised and edited by Dr. Clayton L. Thomas, 1973.

"The Great Con-ola." The Weston A. Price Foundation.

Today's Herbal Health. Louise Tenney, 2000.

Therapeutics Materia Medica and Pharmacy, twelfth edition. Dr. Samuel Potter, 1912.

Understanding Normal and Clinical Nutrition, sixth edition. Wadsworth Eleanor Whitney, Corrine Cataldo, Sharon Rolfes, 2002.

Understanding Normal and Clinical Nutrition, eighth edition. Wadsworth Sharon Rady Rolfes, Kathryn Pinna, Ellie Whitney. 2009.

United States Dispensatory, twelfth edition. 1865.

The United States Dispensatory Pharmacopoeia. Wood & Bache 1865

American Psychological Association APA.org

Centers For Disease Control https://www.atsdr.cdc.gov/emes/public/ docs/Chemicals, Cancer, and You FS.pdf (Drugabuse.gov.)

Centers for Disease Control https://cdc.gov https://www.cdc.gov/nchs/ data/nvsr/nvsr68/nvsr68_06-508.pdf

Risk Factors for Cancer https://www.atsdr.cdc.gov/emes/public/docs/ Chemicals,%20Cancer,%20and%20You%20FS.pdf

https://fulcompany.com

https://www.goodhousekeeping.com/food-recipes/cooking/g532/ types-of-lettuce/

https://laidbackgardener.blog/2019/04/28/ the-mystery-behind-the-garden-huckleberry/

The Institute for Natural Healing https://ethics.harvard.edu/blog/ new-prescription-drugs-major-health-risk-few-offsetting-advantages

https://www.healthline.com/health/ autoimmune-disorders#common-autoimmune-diseases

https://www.healthline.com/nutrition/ why-high-fructose-corn-syrup-is-bad

https://www.hopkinsmedicine.org/

https://shopwondrousroots.com/turkey-rhubarb-root/

https://nida.nih.gov/research-topics/trends-statistics/ overdose-death-rates

https://www.ncbi.nlm.nih.gov/pmc/articles/PMC2571842/pdf/ jnma00292-0091.pdf. https://www.ncbi.nlm.nih.gov/pmc/articles/ PMC4707300/ National Library of Medicine

www.rsc.org Royal Society of Chemistry

https://shirleytwofeathers.com/The_Blog/encyclopediaofherbology/ sample-page/glossary-of-herbal-actions/

https://www.duchessoil.co.uk/news-articles/2016/5/14/
  rapeseed-a-brief-history

https://universityhealthnews.com/daily/nutrition/
  what-does-soda-do-to-your-body/(soda)

https://fullscript.com/blog/excipients

https://www.healthline.com/nutrition/
  why-high-fructose-corn-syrup-is-bad

https://medlineplus.gov/ency/article/000276.htm Lactose Intolerance

https://thegrownetwork.com/how-to-make-an-electuary/

https://www.thespruceeats.com/type-of-oil-for-stir-frying-4077047

https://umasstox.com/2017/02/21/what-is-sassafras/

http://www.hub-uk.com/cooking/tipssassafras.htm

https://www.dvidshub.net/news/416635/sweet-us-troops-have-savored-
  taste-chocolates-their-rations-since-world-war-ii

https://www.planetayurveda.com/sheeps-sorrel-rumex-acetosell

https://dta0yqvfnusiq.cloudfront.net/allnaturalhealingsrq/2019/04/How-
  Rockefeller-Founded-Big-Pharma-and-Waged-War-on-Natural-
  Cures-5cb3d7374f337.pdf

https://www.youtube.com/watch?v=OwMoD3apAQ0 (Dr. Mark
  Hyman/canola oil)

https://www.youtube.com/watch?v=wPlHuXYI8v0 (Dr. Ken Berry/
  canola oil)

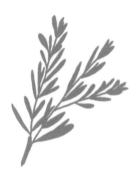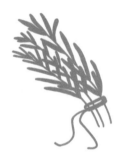

Resources

The American Botanical Council herbalgram.org

In 1988, serious, independent herbalists, scientists, doctors, and industry executives formed this council to set standards, provide information, and debunk myths related to the necessity and efficacy of herbs. Herbalgram's historical and current research are critical to the professional standards of the health food industry. Their founder, Mark Blumenthal, speaks nationally and internationally to schools of medicine, government authorities, academic institutions, and industry symposiums about the importance of plant medicine.

The American Herbalists Guild americanherbalistsguild.com

Since 1989, the guild has been holding conferences, sponsoring workshops, and saluting the important work of ethnobotanists nationally and internationally. With chapters across the United States, herbal practitioners can come together and learn.

The National Health Federation thenhf.com

Since 1955, NHF has been leading the charge to allow private citizens the right to health freedom. Standing up in courts and public forums, NHF has supported people who want to choose the herbs, vitamins, and drugs they will use. Their magazine, *Health Freedom*, is a compendium of current cases here and in Europe where regulating powers are trying to block health freedom rights. Their president, Scott Tips, is on the international roll call of attendees to the World Health Organization's Codex Alimentarius Commission hearings where standards are being set about how herbs and nutraceuticals can be marketed and sold.

United Plant Savers unitedplantsavers.org
Since 1994, this non-profit's mission is to protect native medicinal plants, fungi, and their habitats while ensuring renewable populations for future generations. Begun by the esteemed herbalist Rosemary Gladstar, their statement is *"The work of United Plant Savers involves research, educa-tion, and conservation of native medicinal plants and their habitats."* They *can offer advice on botanical sanctuary networks and planting.*

https://www.starwest-botanicals.com/
A good online source for bulk herbs.

https://mountainroseherbs.com
A good online source for bulk herbs.

https://oregonswildharvest.com
A good online source for bulk herbs.

Sardi, Bill *You Don't Have to Be Afraid of Cancer Anymore.*